LIGHT that HEALS

ENERGY MEDICINE
TODAY & BEYOND

Other books by Donna Fisher

Silent Fields: The Growing Cancer Cluster Story

More Silent Fields: Cancer and the Dirty Electricity Plague

Dirty Electricity and Electromagnetic Radiation:
Understanding Electromagnetic Energy

Praise for *Dirty Electricity and Electromagnetic Radiation*

An important, valuable and compelling book. It may really save your life.

Dr Ross Walker, Cardiologist, Health Ambassador for Asteron Life Insurance,
best-selling author and regarded as one of the world's best keynote speakers.

One of the better books.

Emeritus professor Martin Graham, Electrical Engineering and Computer Science,
University of California, Berkeley, USA

Thank you for this, dear Donna Fisher. I will immediately send the information around! With my very best regards.

Olle Johansson, PhD, Associate Professor of the Experimental Dermatology Unit, Department of
Neuroscience Karolinska Institute, Professor of The Royal Institute of Technology, Stockholm, Sweden

An excellent book which pieces together the big picture related to the public health effects of electrical pollution and transmitted radiofrequency radiation (from wireless technology). It is well worth reading.

Ms Fisher pulls together diverse studies and statistics to support her points. The book makes a strong case that in order to achieve a healthy public, we will need to properly engineer our electrical systems and devices and minimize our use of wireless technology. It is an important read for anyone trying to keep their family safe in our modern world.

For instance, did you know that a study of 44,788 pairs of twins found that environmental effects were responsible for initiating the majority of cancers? Breast cancer, leukemia, and lymphoma all have established links to EMF exposure. Even lung, melanoma, prostate, bladder, and colon cancer seem to be correlated. She also discusses the relationship to autism, ADD/ADHD, SIDS, multiple sclerosis, CFS, fibromyalgia, asthma, diabetes, Alzheimer's disease, etc.

Electrical Pollution Solutions www.electricalpollution.com

LIGHT that HEALS

ENERGY MEDICINE TODAY & BEYOND

Donna Fisher

CARTER
FILM & BOOK PUBLISHING

CARTER
FILM & BOOK PUBLISHING

PUBLISHER	Carter Film & Book Publishing
	PO Box 1027, Runaway Bay 4216 Queensland, Australia
EMAIL	donna@donnafisher.net
WEBSITE	donnafisher.net

LIGHT THAT HEALS - ENERGY MEDICINE, TODAY & BEYOND

National Library of Australia Cataloguing-in-Publication data

AUTHOR	Fisher, Donna, author.
TITLE	Light that heals : energy medicine, today & beyond / Donna Fisher.
ISBN	9780992412906 (paperback) 9781742983783 (eBook)
NOTES	Includes bibliographical references and index.
SUBJECTS	Cancer – Treatment.
	Cancer – Risk factors.
	Electric lines – Health aspects.
	Electromagnetic fields – Health aspects.
	Electromagnetic waves – Health aspects.

DEWEY NUMBER 616.994

EDITOR	Donna Fisher
DESIGN	Graham Rendoth R33037-FA4	www.renodesign.com.au
IMAGES	Various sources, with permission
PRINTING	Lightning Source

DEDICATION

This book is dedicated to the many scientists who work so diligently on their research in the quest to help humanity. It is indeed a humbling experience to be able to spread this information. I have been privileged in that the people dedicated to the research in this area have given me their time and answered my persistent questions, answers to which throw up yet more questions. It is my hope that I have done justice to their work.

ACKNOWLEDGMENTS

Most of all, thank you to my family, who have supported me throughout the writing of all of my books. To my friends and colleagues who read my manuscript, I greatly appreciate your suggestions.

I extend special thanks to Graham Rendoth of Reno Design, for his design and publishing expertise. Suggestions on the title of the book resulted in more extensive research into 'light'. His direction, patience and caring attitude to the content has resulted in a much improved and extended version of the original transcript.

I would like to thank Dr Charles and Linda Neophytou for their unswerving support and for publishing my first book, *Silent Fields*. I also thank John and Cheryl Bannister from Joshua Books for supporting me throughout my writing and for publishing *More Silent Fields* and *Dirty Electricity and Electromagnetic Radiation*. I would also like to thank Michelle Holyhead of The Book Studio, Australia for her expertise and attention to detail.

Thank you to those who, when I lecture, stand up and robustly challenge me while I am imparting the information on dirty electricity. Their resistance to what is relatively new information has energized me to research even deeper into areas which have also challenged my own beliefs.

CONTENTS

FOREWORD

I am both proud and honored to write the foreword for Donna's latest book. We first met when I read her first book as our small coastal town was threatened by a second mobile phone tower. Her book helped raise community awareness about potential harm from some of the electromagnetic spectrum. Eventually, with our local Federal MP Janelle Saffi's help, the tower did not eventuate. It is interesting to note that our concerns have now been vindicated in a recent study from Israel showing the harm from living within 400 metres of a mobile phone tower.

I have read Donna's latest books and as Samuel Milham told her, 'tell anyone who will listen that dirty electricity is causing cancer'. This is what I now do at every opportunity.

Donna may not fully appreciate the great help she has provided people with her efforts. The public awareness regarding potential harm from some EMF frequencies is growing rapidly and hopefully one day public opinion will win out.

Professionally I see the harm done to patients on a daily basis. I have been a GP here for 13 years and our previous very low cancer rate has skyrocketed in the past 12 months or so. At one stage I was seeing one new case per week. Of even greater concern is most of these are in two parallel streets: one contains our only mobile phone tower that has been upgraded to 4G and most of these patients live within 400 metres.

The only other changes I have seen are related to the massively increased dirty electricity upgrade in power supply into town and the uptake of solar that creates dirty electricity when converting DC power to AC. Can I prove my supposition, of course not, but I personally measure levels of dirty electricity and have noticed consistent levels above 2000 GS units. These levels were not noted when Donna first came to our town in 2008. Our only primary school had levels over 2000 GS units in multiple rooms. Fortunately the school has now been filtered with noticeable changes in children's behavior.

Unfortunately common sense has not prevailed and in order to 'keep up with technology', they have now against my advice installed WiFi. Apparently the Education Department does not see this as an issue. Of even greater concern is this system apparently cannot be turned off and now irradiates the closest neighbours even when school is out.

Personally I think Donna should change writing genre to Medical or Legal

Fiction or even to Science Fiction. Imagine the stories she could write about: growing cancer clusters, dirty electricity, inappropriate standards, electricity, WiFi, autism, ADHD, and type 3 diabetes. I await the day the legal profession catches on.

Donna's books are possibly not going to be No.1 Best Sellers, for despite their worldwide relevance, people can too easily ignore the messages. It would be totally different if the harmful frequencies could be seen. Unfortunately in years to come, the harm will be obvious but too late for many, and those involved will pretend they didn't know.

Donna's latest work expands initially on her very impressive knowledge, with more detail about harm but then concludes with some wonderful information about light that heals.

I think like me, you will be impressed by her work. I remain proud, honored and very impressed. I think you will be too.

Dr David Richards MBBS, FACRRM

INTRODUCTION

As we go further into the future, the legends of Atlantis will become more of a reality, when we live in a world where our lighting will be glowing crystals and our pain and suffering is alleviated by wands of light. Light devices will replace scalpels, acupuncture needles will be replaced by needles of light, chemotherapy will be replaced by phototherapy and prescription drugs by prescription colors. As we continue to utilize light technologies, cancer may soon become a disease of the past.

On this amazing journey of knowledge and wisdom, I traveled to Heliopolis, originally called On (City of Light), in Egypt, where it is believed the first Sun Temple in the Western world was constructed. Then on to Alexandria where the Ancient Therapeutae lived, as Alexandria replaced Heliopolis as the centre of Sun worship. I was then led to the USA where my personal energetic imprint was taken by a technology based on NASA research. If I develop a health challenge in the future, I was advised my energetic signature can be assessed and a vibrational signature sent to me in Australia.

I have investigated and witnessed many interesting treatments from those working with light and energy across different countries and cultures. The wide-ranging spectrum of 'healing' therapies is an intriguing area, and some therapies continue to challenge my beliefs. One such experience is when I underwent 'Crystal Bed' therapy where I laid on a table with seven different colored crystals suspended above me with pulsating lights shining through. This led me to investigate color therapy further, and ultimately include a chapter on colors, crystals and chakras.

It has been through my research for this book that I fully comprehended the uniqueness of the capsules that I had ingested daily for 14 years. These capsules contained a physical substance and a concentrated form of 'life sustaining' energy within them. Unfortunately, this creation is now not available and 'lost' to the world.

On believing I had completed this book, my son urged me to watch the movie *Elysium*, where a girl in the final stages of leukemia is returned to a state of health, when her body is 're-atomized' after being placed under a light technology that scans her body. My son's suggestion to find out if this can really be possible, led me through a series of synchronistic events.

I had been gifted another EMF protection device so I decided to gift it to a woman I had been trying to assist for many years who was particularly sensitive to artificial electromagnetic fields (EMF). She said she did not need any other product, as on purchasing two BLUSHIELD devices that gave out a scalar field, she was no longer affected by this electromagnetic pollution. Previous to this, she felt to find peace, she would have to live 'away from the things of man' in a forest or in a protected area in Sweden, as she had become very debilitated from being exposed to this electromagnetic pollution which few today can escape.

Catherine stated: 'It is a miracle, I am no longer affected by EMF.' I found this remarkable. As I do not feel the effects from these fields immediately myself, but know that they are still harming me, I then trialled a BLUSHIELD Tesla device with a building biologist who was also debilitated from these fields. She was so amazed at the result she did not want to return the product. It is the individuals who alert us to the effects of these fields who can also guide us as to how to protect ourselves from these fields.

I then found it particularly interesting that one of the first doctors to arouse suspicion, as he was affected by these fields and then went on to test his patients, Dr William Rea, stated: 'It appears that the body is responding to the BLUSHIELD allowing the body to ignore more stressful environmental frequencies emitted from electrical devices, including mobile phones.'

It is my understanding that the body recognizes and resonates with the field, designed on natural laws and mathematical principles that BLUSHIELD technology emits, thus creating an environment to override harmful EMF. The body will always favor fields that act in accordance with natural laws pertaining to body systems and the body's natural rhythms and cycles.

On being introduced to the world of scalar energy, I then entered a specially designed chamber utilizing the Energy Enhancement System (EES), which generates a therapeutic energy field known by physicists as scalar waves. Even though eight computers were emanating scalar waves I was to learn that scalar energy overrides the harmful effects of EMF.

That same day I also underwent a Physiospect Non-Linear Analysis. Via specially designed headphones, this technology sends an infrared triggering signal to the bio-field around the brain where I witnessed in real time on a computer screen, the health status of my entire body – organs, tissues, cells, all components down to 197 segments of DNA that make up the genes in the chromosomes and also some neurotransmitters and hormones. Seeing the condition of my body's bio-field (the 'aura') was fascinating.

What was so intriguing is the corrective procedure termed META-Therapy. With the push of a button, I saw the disturbed frequency patterns of the areas that were scanned being corrected. It was like defragging a computer from the corruptions gathered through the process of living. I was advised this correction, occurring initially at the blueprint level, is a true quantum therapy that immediately initiates the repair process in the energetic realm. In the quest to achieve a state of optimal functioning, further visits and other measures are required.

I was then prompted to order James Oschman's book, *Energy Medicine: The Scientific Basis*, in which he states scalar waves appear to interact with atomic nuclei. Re-atomizing the body and atomic nuceli in the body being affected. Another 'aha' moment. On finally sourcing the Element 5, a scalar wave technology, I am in awe of what one day will be. The concept of reprogramming the human matrix to a coherent state of optimal functioning is no longer magical thinking.

Light that Heals is the result of my research from being thrown into darkness when I believed the lives of my family and I would be put at risk.

My first book, *Silent Fields: The Growing Cancer Cluster Story – When Electricity Kills*, still stands on its own, written due to the inadequate investigation of the electrical environment into a workplace breast cancer cluster. It is an exposé on the power industry, detailing the lead-up to the court case, the court case that created a world-first, and the surprising lawyers and expert witnesses involved.

Just as this book was about to be printed I was alerted to the release of a ground-breaking study of a cancer cluster at a school in California where dirty electricity was implicated, so I swiftly added a chapter on dirty electricity and filters that removed dirty electricity. On reading *Silent Fields: The Growing Cancer Cluster Story – When Electricity Kills*, a building biologist contacted me and advised how her health had improved when the dirty electricity levels were lowered in her home and workplace.

I immediately contacted Dave Stetzer, who co-created the filters, and he provided me with even more startling information which I could not ignore. Experiencing trouble getting his dirty electricity levels down in his home, Stetzer had asked his neighbors who were on the same transformer if he could place filters to remove the dirty electricity in their home. He did this on a Wednesday night. It just so happened that the lady of the house had been diagnosed that day with leukemia. She went back the next Monday to a specialist to determine the best procedure to attack the disease, but her blood had cleared up in about five days. That was in 1998 and she is fine today with no treatments for leukemia.

At the same time, Stetzer went to another neighboring home on the same transformer and also installed filters. The couple there were in their 40s and had no children. Following installation of the filters, the woman became ill at times. On seeing several doctors, she was advised she was pregnant and attributes her pregnancy to the removal of dirty electricity by the filters, as it was the only change in her environment. The woman worked at a courthouse where there were a lot of energy efficient lights, computers and general electronic equipment, which are known to contribute to dirty electricity.

Around this time, an Australian legal case uncovered that a USA power company had observed that two girls who had powerlines running very close to their homes had developed breast cancer at a particularly early age.

Furthering my research I was to meet a man whose multiple sclerosis went into remission twelve months after removing dirty electricity from his home, a building biologist whose health improved dramatically from also removing dirty electricity from her home. I was given a testimony from a man who had the dirty electricity removed from his home and noticed improvements in his son who had autism. He also found he no longer suffered headaches. What was going on?

All this information prompted me to continue my investigation of the scientific, medical and electrical worlds. So I kept up the challenging task to research and distribute this information through publishing books.

However, after 14 years of research and writing on the artificial electro-magnetic fields (EMF) that emanate from our electrical wiring, I was to dis-cover that EMF when uncontrolled can harm, and when controlled, can heal. My second book *More Silent Fields: Cancer and the Dirty Electricity Plague – The Missing Link* and my third book *Dirty Electricity and Electromagnetic Radiation: Understanding Electromagnetic Energy* discussed EMF that can harm and touched on the EMF being used to heal.

On receiving photodynamic therapy for a skin cancer that left no scarring, I was introduced to the world of 'light'. I was to discover that light enters the eyes, not only to serve vision, but to go directly to the body's biological clock within the hypothalamus. The hypothalamus controls the nervous system and endocrine system, whose combined effects regulate all biological functions in humans.

As physicists often refer to all electromagnetic phenomena as 'light', I have included the information from my second and third books. This new book, *Light that Heals*, enables the reader to have such wide-ranging information available in a single source.

You will discover it is believed that the brain perceives the artificial EMF that permeates our lives on a daily basis as 'light'. I put forward the sugges-tion that we are suffering from misillumination, that these artificial EMF are affecting the light in our bodies at the energetic level.

This book is a result of conversations with numerous doctors, therapists and lay persons. In regard to the technologies I refer to, they are supplied for the reader to further understand electromagnetic energy as they are the ones I came across in my research. I do not have endorsement contracts with any product and I have not been paid to promote any device. There are also many other devices available that stem from the information in this book.

As much as we seek to eliminate and alleviate pain and suffering, engaging in preventative strategies today is essential. In February 2014, the International Agency for Research on Cancer (IARC) – the cancer agency for the World Health Organization (WHO) – presented the *World Cancer Report 2014*, a collaboration of over 250 leading scientists from more than 40 countries. Dr Christopher Wild PhD and professor Bernard Stewart announced we must focus on prevention on a massive scale, as cancer rates are growing at such a rapid pace that we cannot treat our way out of this global health crisis: in 2012, the worldwide burden of cancer rose to an estimated 14 million new cases per year, a figure expected to rise to 22 million annually within the next two decades.

With the increase in non-invasive electromagnetic energy treatments and more orthodox methods becoming individual and target specific, physically aggressive methods will become less of a reality. It is my hope that physically aggressive behaviors will also lessen as we strive to consciously go toward the light and become ultimately harmless.

'All truth passes through three stages: First, it is ridiculed; Second, it is violently opposed; and Third, it is accepted as self-evident.'

Arthur Schopenhauer (1788–1860)

PART 1

LIGHT THAT HARMS

01

THE UNDERLYING
MENACE EXPOSED

*'... chronic exposure to these fields is a competent
cause for the origin of cancers.'*

Dr Robert O Becker – *The Body Electric*, 1990

Last century, we should have become healthier due to improved hygiene practices and medical advancements. However, we descended into a civilization where so many different diseases developed and millions have died from cancer or are living with cancer.

In November 2009, a ground-breaking study on the history of electrification of the USA was published. Professor of Medicine Dr Samuel Milham MPH and one-time chief epidemiologist at the Washington State Health Department, USA, researched when 48 states of the USA were electrified. He also compared the urban populations that lived with electricity and the rural areas which did not have electricity, which led to his discovery that most of the twentieth century diseases of civilization, including cancer, cardiovascular disease, diabetes and suicide are caused by exposure to the fields emanating from electrical wiring – electromagnetic fields (EMF).[1]

Due to his position and having access to all the statistics in the land, Milham states that the health and mortality effects of electrification happened so gradually and on such a wide scale, that they went virtually unnoticed, and the major illnesses that can be attributed to them came to be considered 'normal' diseases of modern civilization. Milham stated in the study: '... it seems unbelievable that mortality differences of this magnitude could go unexplained for over 70 years after they were first reported and 40 years after they were noticed.' In his book *Dirty Electricity: Electrification and the Diseases of Civilization*, he comments: 'The data to prove this has been available since 1930 but no one investigated it.'

Milham reports that since 1900 there has been a gradual increase in mortality rates of cancer, cardiovascular disease, diabetes and suicide, the so-called diseases of civilization. This is in sharp contrast to the gradual decline in the death rate from all causes, which was reflecting increasing control of infectious diseases. Since 1900, heart disease has been the number one killer in the USA every year except 1918, the year of the great influenza epidemic.[2]

Milham also brings attention to a community-based epidemiologic study in the mid-1980s of urban and rural differences in coronary heart disease and its risk factors, carried out in New Delhi, India and in a rural area 50 kilometers away.[3] The prevalence of coronary heart disease was three times higher in the urban residents, despite the fact that the rural residents smoked more and had higher total caloric and saturated fat intakes. Most cardiovascular disease risk factors were two to three times more common in the urban residents. Rural electrification projects are still being carried out in parts of the rural area that was studied.

Dr Michael Court-Brown and epidemiologist Richard Doll reported as early as 1960 that a new leukemia agent was introduced into the UK and USA in the 1920s and 1930s. In 2001, Milham, while working with the Washington State Department of Health, completed a study with E M Ossiander on the history of electrification of the UK and USA. They concluded that the childhood leukemia peak of (cALL) was attributable to residential electrification: 75 percent of all childhood acute lymphoblastic leukemia and 60 percent of all childhood leukemia could be preventable.[4]

While conducting this ground-breaking study, Milham noticed a strong positive correlation between residential electrification and mortality for some adult cancers, including female breast cancers, in the 1930 and 1940 vital statistics. He found that 1930 urban cancer death rates were 58.8 percent higher than rural cancer death rates where there was no electricity. Rural death rates were significantly correlated with the level of residential electric service by state for most of the causes examined.[5]

The Ashkenazi Jewish population has assisted in the study of hereditary breast/ovarian cancer syndrome, caused by mutations in the BRCA1 and BRCA2 genes, and the Finnish population in hereditary nonpolyposis colorectal cancer (HNPCC) caused by MLH1 gene mutations.[6] Neither of the above-mentioned two groups though has retained the unique lifestyle of the Amish as, unlike the Amish, neither has remained isolated in the post-industrial revolution era.

The Amish of Holmes County Ohio are the largest Amish population in the world and a recent study by an Ohio State University Medical Center Group concluded cancer incidence is low in the Ohio Amish, based on data which cannot be explained solely on the basis of their tobacco abstinence or other factors.[7]

The Amish live without electricity, especially the Old Order Amish (OOA). The Amish in the USA and Canada who live without electricity have a current pattern of morbidity and mortality similar to that of USA rural residents in the early part of the 20th century who also lived without electricity. At the turn of the 20th century, when almost all USA cities were electrified, urban residents had an average life expectancy below 50 years. The life expectancy of the Amish though is above 70 years and has been stable since 1890. The OOA have had a life expectancy of about 72 years for the past 300 years for both men and women.[8]

Like rural USA residents in the 1940s, Amish males in the 1970s had very low cancer and cardiovascular disease mortality rates.[9] The Amish that have been studied also have decreased rates of breast and prostate cancers.[10] Alzheimer's disease has also been reported to have a low prevalence in the Amish.[11]

A pediatric group practice in Jasper, Indiana, which cares for more than 800 Amish families, has not diagnosed a single child in this group with attention deficit hyperactivity disorder (ADHD).[12] Childhood obesity is also virtually non-existent in this population. The Amish type 2 diabetes prevalence rates are about half those of the non-Amish, even though their obesity rates are comparable.

The generation of electricity in the final years of the 1800s would usher in a new way of living, which would eventually enable us to live 24-hour days in artificial light and artificially created EMF.

However, with this new way of living, there was also a dramatic change in the way we live – a new plague, silent and invisible, that would spread far and wide over the planet, bringing with it many of the so-called diseases of civilization.

The plague of Dirty Electricity

The previous and other current plagues in history will pale in comparison to the current dirty electricity plague that gained momentum at the beginning of last century and virtually went unnoticed for 100 years.

Due to the very nature of how electricity is delivered 'dirty electricity' – Transient EMF – has existed from the first generation of electricity.[13] Dirty electricity is also described as Electrical Pollution and Harmonic Pollution by the electrical industry, a term which can also be used for describing its effects on the body.

Our brain, our heart and the trillions of cells in our bodies depend on sending and receiving naturally produced electric and electromagnetic signals and it is crucial that this process is not altered or damaged, as every biochemical process involves the precisely choreographed movement of EMF-sensitive atoms, molecules and ions.

It appears that the body recognizes EMF as a foreign invader and mounts an acute stress response to it. With chronic exposure and stress, neuroendocrine and immune system dysregulation results in a wide spectrum of human morbidity and mortality. In 1955, Dr Hans Seyle – considered the father of stress research – explained how chronic stress leads to disease.[14]

Every thought, action, and emotion involves communications between brain cells that are triggered by special chemicals called neurotransmitters. It is now generally accepted that most mental disorders involve imbalanced levels or altered functioning of these critically important brain chemicals.

Milham posits dirty electricity, and probably other types of EMF exposures, act as chronic stressors causing neurotransmitter changes and disease. Milham states that evidence that neurotransmitter abnormalities are associated with disease are, the number of conditions for which drugs targeting neurotransmitters are used. These include, but are not limited to: depression, ADHD, schizophrenia, Parkinson's disease, restless leg syndrome, eating disorders, anxiety disorders, insomnia and chronic fatigue syndrome.[15]

In 2012, it was shown that neurotransmitters and dopamine levels leave the body when exposed to dirty electricity. Milham posits neurotransmitters may be biomarkers of dirty electricity and EMF exposures.[16] Our neurotransmitters – molecules that transmit information from one nerve cell to another – are the electrical grid in the body for the immune system. It is how the immune system communicates with the brain. If they are not there, the signals get interrupted and the immune system does not work in the way it is supposed to.

It is believed artificial EMF are perceived by the brain as 'light'. When light enters the eye, some 20 percent of it carries on past the retina and reaches vital components of the brain, especially the hypothalamus, the pituitary gland and the pineal gland, the body's light meter. By this means, light (and by implication all kinds of EMF) can regulate the majority of our life processes, including hormone production, stress response, the autonomic nervous system, and the limbic system that is the seat of our emotions. Apart from these, the light – once inside us – can affect our metabolism and even our reproductive functions.[17]

Dr Jacob Liberman, in his book *Light: Medicine of the Future*, reports that each eye contains 137 million photoreceptors – approximately 130 million photoreceptors called rods and 7 million called cones – which transform light into electrical impulses that are then sent to the brain at approximately 234 miles per hour.

Life is also bound by the unhindered and unaltered free-flowing information sequences within our bodies, so that the electromagnetic signature of cells, tissues and organs maintain their precise and intricate actions and reactions, responses and adjustments.

02

ELECTRICITY AND DISEASE

'New research is suggesting that nearly all the human plagues which emerged in the twentieth century, like common acute lymphoblastic leukemia in children, female breast cancer, malignant melanoma and asthma, can be tied to some facet of our use of electricity.'

Samuel Milham, MD, MPH – Washington State Department of Health, USA 2008

The premise that the silent and invisible EMF from electricity could kill, and make others very sick, has been met with disbelief, yet many people unable to trace the cause of their illnesses finally find relief when exposure to these fields created from electricity is lessened.

In 2007, in the *Journal of the Royal Institute of Public Health*, independent researcher on electromagnetic radiation Dr Stephen J Genuis, Faculty of Medicine, University of Alberta in Canada, highlights the following case studies:[1]

CASE HISTORY 1

A 66-year-old woman in generally good health complained of a nine-year history of debilitating daily headaches and intermittent dizziness. Neurological assessment was unremarkable and a computer tomography scan, magnetic resonance imaging and electroencephalogram were reported normal.

At a chronic-pain clinic, the patient received narcotic analgesics and a diagnosis of 'primary pain disorder'. Detailed aetiological history was unremarkable, other than the patient used an electric toothbrush six times a day for meticulous care of failing dentition. Gaussmeter assessment revealed inordinately high levels of EMFs (≥200 mG units) emanating from the toothbrush. Within six weeks of discontinuing the use of her toothbrush, the headaches subsided and, with assistance, she was quickly able to overcome her dependence on prescription analgesics.

CASE HISTORY 2

A 33-year-old woman wishing to have a large family complained of six consecutive pregnancy losses. After two uncomplicated pregnancies with vaginal deliveries, the patient changed residences and subsequently experienced three first-trimester miscarriages.

After assessments by a family physician, a gynaecologist, an infertility specialist and a specialty reproductive care unit, the patient subsequently sustained three second-trimester losses despite interventions, including clomiphene, human chorionic gonadotrophin injections, progesterone supplementation and counselling. According to her history, the only potential determinant that appeared to have changed from when she experienced the two completed gestations was her employment as a seamstress for six hours a day in the basement of her new residence, an environment with low ceilings and fluorescent lights.

Using a gaussmeter, the woman recorded high EMF levels (≥ 104 mG units) in the vicinity of her head when fluorescent lighting in her workplace was turned on, and high EMF levels (~180 mG units) adjacent to her sewing machine. Following advice to decrease EMR exposure by avoiding fluorescent lights and minimising the use of her sewing machine, the woman promptly conceived and carried the pregnancy to full term.

CASE HISTORY 3

A 17-year-old boy experiencing a three-year history of intrusive thoughts relating to religious themes believed he had committed unpardonable sins and was convinced the devil was imminently sending him to hell. As well as increasing depressive symptoms, the adolescent displayed escalating aggression towards his parents. The nominally religious parents took their son for religious counselling, to no avail. Psychiatric diagnosis included a thought disorder. Psychotropic medication failed to control the symptoms but caused numerous side effects.

Human exposure assessment uncovered extremely high gauss measurements (≥ 200 mG units) at the head of the teen's bed, as electrical entry to the house was immediately adjacent to the bedroom, right beside his bed. He moved to another bedroom and all other sources of EMF exposure were minimized.

Within twelve weeks, the intrusive thoughts had abated considerably, the mood symptomatology had declined, medication was stopped, and the parents indicated that their son was now a friendly, motivated boy. One episode of symptom aggravation subsequently occurred immediately following four hours of online work in a high school computer laboratory, those symptoms subsided within seventy-two hours of deliberate EMF avoidance. All adverse symptoms completely cleared within six months and wellness was maintained over the next two years and at the time of writing.

EMF – electric and magnetic fields – are produced wherever electricity is generated, transmitted or used. The above three examples discuss the magnetic field – mG unit measurements.

The EMF we are exposed to emanate from powerlines, substations, wiring in buildings, electrical appliances and equipment (e.g. hairdryers, alarm clocks, refrigerators, microwaves, computers, photo-developing machines, hospital equipment, baby monitors, humidicribs). EMF appears to be affecting our neurochemistry in far reaching ways.

The late Dr Neil Cherry, when associate professor at Lincoln University, New Zealand traveled the world visiting the research clinics to collate all the data. He concluded that EMF affect the brain's melatonin/serotonin homeostasis that is vital for our physical, mental and emotional health.

Lessening exposure to EMF

Consider a vulnerable child with or recovering from leukemia – in fact any person with cancer – in hospital being exposed to high measurements of these silent EMF from medical equipment and wiring while they are awake and particularly, as they sleep.

Consider a child at school or a person spending long hours in their workplace where the fluorescent lighting and wiring from the floor below are emitting high measurements of these silent EMF beneath them.

Consider people sleeping with the meter box on the other side of their bedroom wall or those who sleep with electrical equipment close to their heads. Consider a transformer outside one's home. Promotional signs directly outside one's apartment or bedroom window can also yield high measurements of EMF.

Exposure to these silent fields, combined with other toxic agents, appears to produce a deadly cocktail. In 2006, an analysis of 65 studies reported that compared to exposure to the toxic agent alone, the combined effect of toxic agents and these silent fields enhanced the damage.[2]

For example, consider a hairdresser who is exposed to chemicals – some of which may contain toxic agents – and who uses a hairdryer for a large part of the day. Although the client is sitting down, the hairdresser is standing and holding at breast level a hairdryer that emits very high measurements of these fields. If a measurement of 1.8 mG units has been indicated with childhood leukemia, what might the average hairdryer, which emits 70 mG units, do?

As another example of the danger of the combined effects of EMF and possibly toxic agents, consider a pregnant female who stands in front of a photo-copying or photo-developing machine for many hours a day, where exposure to high measurements of EMF should be of concern. Now consider the effect of EMF exposure combined with potential toxic chemicals emitted from the machine.

The smoking link

Consider people who smoke. The chemical carcinogens in cigarette smoke cause 'DNA breaks' that damage our precious and life-giving DNA. Damaged DNA increases the risk of cancer.

Similarly, exposure to EMF has also been shown to cause DNA breaks.[3] So if you are a smoker, being exposed to both is a double hit. Cigarette-smoking and EMF can both damage DNA on their own. EMF can also enhance the toxic exposure from the cigarettes. Also, mobile phone radiation has been found to amplify the DNA damage caused by a chemical mutagen.[4]

In January 2009, scientists at the Cancer Institute NSW in Australia, found that leukemia, brain, kidney and eye cancers are common in children whose mothers smoked during pregnancy, drawing for the first time a direct link with cancer. The Institute linked the records of all births in New South Wales between 1994 and 2005 with causes of cancer in children during the same period. Even though smoking during pregnancy has long been advised against, scientists have never before drawn a direct link with cancer.

Will it also take decades before the wisdom of avoiding direct exposure to EMF while pregnant is common knowledge?

Cause and effect

When a report by the California Department of Health Services was released in 2002, legal counsel for the electrical industry worldwide conceded that the attitude of the power industry had to change. The belief of legal representatives for the power industry was that it would be 'legally inadvisable' to make a global statement that there is no cause-and-effect relationship between these fields and disease.[5] This privileged Attorney-Client Communication, supplied in Appendix A, was obtained in a legal manner.

The Russians commenced addressing measures to protect their citizens from these EMF since the 1950s and the Swedish government instigated measures in the 1990s. Denmark, Italy, Switzerland, Israel, the Netherlands and Slovenia are also in the process of implementing measures.

ELF EMF (extremely low frequency) exposures were classified as an IARC 2B (possible) carcinogen in 2001.[6] This addresses the magnetic field. In June 2007, the WHO concluded that reducing exposure to EMF from power exposure is reasonable and warranted, provided that the health, social and economic benefits of electric power are not compromised.[7]

Another side to electricity

In 2007, Genuis addresses dirty electricity in the *Journal of the Royal Institute of Public Health*. The fourth case studied was:

CASE HISTORY 4

A 51-year-old man in generally good health complained of chronic difficulty with insomnia. Although he experienced no problem falling asleep, for the last 17 years he had routinely awoken at about 2:30 am after 4 hours of slumber and was consistently unable to return to sleep. As a result of sleep deprivation, he experienced constant fatigue, often falling asleep at various intervals during the day. While on holiday in their mobile home, however, the patient enjoyed improved sleep, causing his physician to attribute the insomnia to job stress. Numerous therapies had been unsuccessful including counselling, relaxation techniques, benzodiazepine medication, acupuncture and various nutritional supplements.

Microsurge meter assessment in the patient's bedroom revealed power surges reaching 1600 GS units (safe levels reported as ≤30 GS units). Filtration of dirty electricity reduced levels to under 30 GS units, and the patient noticed a dramatic and consistent improvement in sleep patterns within 1 week.[8]

Dirty electricity, another facet of electricity that is proving to be more perilous and more prevalent in our lives, is an invisible and unwelcome character that relies on an unchecked and already overloaded power system.

The pioneer who cautioned on EMF, Dr Robert O Becker, believed the increasing proliferation of EMF to be a greater threat than global warming. EMF from electricity so concerned him that in 1990 he stated:

> … it is quite possible that chronic exposure to these fields is a competent cause for the origin of cancers. This is compatible with the latest data indicating significant increases in the incidence of specific types of cancers since 1975.

According to Dr Samuel Epstein of the University of Chicago Medical Center:

- lymphoma, myeloma, and melanoma have increased by 100 percent
- breast cancer by 31 percent
- cancer of the kidney by 142 percent
- colon cancer by 63 percent [9]

In regard to children, alarmingly, acute lymphoblastic leukemia (ALL) in boys and girls increased 27 percent between 1973 and 1990. Since then, the rate in boys has declined, though it is still rising in girls. Brain cancer increased nearly 40 percent from 1973 to 1994. Brain cancers and other tumors in children's nervous systems rose by more than 25 percent between 1973 and 1996. [10]

What had happened to create such a dramatic rise in cancers? One very important event that had significant influence in our world occurred in the early 1970s.

During the oil embargo of 1973, manufacturers of equipment were forced to design products that would save energy. One method was to have the equipment draw current in an intermittent way (short pulses of current) instead of in a continuous flow. Unfortunately this created overloading of our wiring, resulting in the 'burning buildings' of the late 1970s and 1980s. The excess current on wiring that was not designed to handle this load caused fires. Because of this change in the mode of flow – going from a continuous to an intermittent electrical flow – something significant occurred.

Even though dirty electricity has existed since the early generation of electricity, this change created dirty electricity en masse, resulting in people being exposed to much higher levels of dirty electricity. The incidence of breast cancer has also increased dramatically since the arrival of these higher levels of dirty electricity.

Dirty electricity is unwanted and undesirable radio frequency (RF) radiation (radio frequencies/radiowaves) running along potentially all electrical wiring both inside and outside buildings. Dirty electricity is also referred to as transients and Transient EMF. The electrical industry refers to these transients as 'dirty power'.

Milham comments that it is possible for some of the effects attributed to the magnetic fields from electricity to come from these transients. Transient EMF, together with the escalation of other cancers and diseases would explain to a large extent the dramatic rise in breast cancer, the dramatic rise in diabetes, the sudden appearance of chronic fatigue syndrome (CFS) and more people experiencing electrohypersensitivity (EHS-sensitivity to electromagnetic radiation).

Transient EMF – another environmental assault that is woven into our societal structure – is a large part of the growing cancer and cancer cluster story.

The International Conference on Electromagnetic Fields and Human Health was held in the Republic of Kazakhstan in September 2003. In November of the same year, the state health department of the Republic of Kazakhstan issued sanitary norms addressing Transient EMF, a move which historically takes decades.[11] The document is provided in Appendix B.

The Republic of Kazakhstan has acknowledged that there is no safe level of exposure to dirty electricity. A limit of 50 GS units (industrial) was immediately mandated to protect workers. For the public, in their homes and non-industrial workplaces, a reading less than 30 GS units is easier to achieve.

The Russian space program, based in the Republic of Kazakhstan, has enabled Kazakhstan to quickly address this issue, as their scientists understand electromagnetic energy. They foresee what the dramatic impact on the health of its citizens will be, immediately and downstream.

On April 25, 2011 the IEEE, the world's largest professional association advancing technology for humanity, announced that the IEEE Standards Association (IEEE-SA) Standards Board approved two new projects to develop standards that will limit the injection of harmonic frequencies (Transient EMF) into the public electric transmission system.[12]

Finally, this is a serious public health issue whose time has come. As Shakespeare stated, 'truth is the daughter of time'.

Australian landmark case, 2013

In a decision handed down February 28, 2013 between Commonwealth Scientific and Industrial Research Organisation (CSIRO) senior research scientist Alexander McDonald and Comcare, a statutory authority of the Australian Federal Government, Comcare is liable to pay to Dr McDonald compensation in accordance with the Safety, Rehabilitation and Compensation Act 1988 (Cth) in respect of an injury, being an aggravation of a condition of nausea, disorientation and headaches and also in respect of an injury, being a chronic adjustment disorder with depressed moods. McDonald experienced symptoms of EMF sensitivity for many years before being diagnosed in 1993. This landmark case was regarding his exposure to EMF in his workplace.[13]

Counsel for the Applicant – Ms C Serpell.

Solicitors for the Applicant – Ryan Carlisle Thomas.

03

CANCER AND
DIRTY ELECTRICITY

'I have no doubt in my mind that at the present time that the greatest polluting element in the Earth's environment is the proliferation of electromagnetic fields. I consider that to be far greater on a global scale than warming ...'

Dr Robert O Becker – *The Body Electric*, 1990

When two highly qualified leaders in their fields came out of retirement due to their concern for the people, new information worthy of creating a paradigm shift emerged. Even though the school district administration had refused a number of requests for these men to assist in the evaluation of a larger number of cancers reported by the teachers at La Quinta Middle School in California, a teacher, Gayle Cohen invited these experts to visit the school after hours to take measurements of the electrical environment, which they did at their own expense.

When these researchers reported their findings to the superintendent of schools, the highly esteemed doctor was threatened with prosecution for 'unlawful ... trespass' and the teacher received a letter of reprimand.

These brave men had honourable intentions and impressive credentials. Winner of the prestigious Ramazzini Award, Samuel Milham, who has investigated over 100 cancer clusters, was the first to link workers exposed to EMF with higher rates of leukemia in 1982. Lloyd Morgan BS, an electronics engineer and a devoted pioneer in brain tumor research in regard to EMF, had been Director of the Central Brain Tumor Registry of the USA.

The teachers then filed a California OSHA complaint that ultimately led to the California Department of Health Services' involvement. The department measured the magnetic field (mG units) and dirty electricity (GS units) levels at the school, providing the exposure data for the La Quinta study. The courageous actions of these people and the interpretation of the data resulted in further validation of the culprit.

A 1994 study of Canadian and French utility workers furnished a tantalizing clue about the carcinogenicity of transients. The study, sponsored by Hydro Quebec, showed a 15-fold increased risk of lung cancer in workers exposed to pulsed high frequency fields, with a rising incidence according to dose. Risk ratios this high, are almost never seen in studies using magnetic fields as a metric. These findings were independent of the smoking status of a worker. Unfortunately Hydro Quebec sequestered the data and disappeared the Positron meter used to make the exposure measurements,[1] so no replication or follow-up was possible by anyone else.[2] The culprit – Transient EMF – was not welcome due to the enormous implications it had for society regarding cancer and increasing disease.

La Quinta Middle School – Landmark cancer cluster study

Earlier studies on the effects of dirty electricity and human health conducted by associate professor Dr Magda Havas of Environmental and Resource Studies, Trent University, Ontario, Canada were pivotal to the investigation of the cancer cluster at La Quinta Middle School, resulting in the groundbreaking study released in 2008. In the years 1988-2005, 137 teachers were employed at the school. On investigating the 18 cancers in these teachers, it was found there was a 1:10,000 possibility that this was due to chance. There were nearly three times more cancer cases than expected. The 18 cancers in the 16 affected teachers were:

- four malignant melanomas
- two female breast cancers
- two cancers of the thyroid
- two uterine cancers
- one Burkitt's lymphoma
- one polycythemia vera (PCV)
- one multiple myeloma
- one leiomyosarcoma
- one cancer of the colon
- one cancer of the pancreas
- one cancer of the larynx

The critical finding was that the authors reported that the cancer incidence in the teachers at this school was unusually high and was strongly associated with dirty electricity. When I asked Milham why this study in the prestigious *American Journal of Industrial Medicine* stated that the cancer incidence was 'strongly associated' with dirty electricity and not caused by dirty electricity, he commented that certain circumstances prevented the term 'caused the cancers' being used: the heat came from 'above' and journal editors don't like the words 'caused cancer' being used. Milham advised: you tell anyone who will listen to you that transients are causing cancer.

The authors stated that dirty electricity may be a universal carcinogen similar to ionizing radiation which is an established cause of cancer. Studies into ionizing radiation have shown an increased incidence in a number of different cancers. What is important is the study at La Quinta Middle School also showed an increase in the number of different cancers.

Milham reports that it was obvious that three years at La Quinta Middle School was enough time and exposure to cause cancer both in the teachers and students.[3]

What is most important is that the cancer risks at La Quinta Middle School are comparable to the cigarette smoking/lung cancer risks, especially as there is no unexposed population.[4]

The authors noted that the relatively short latency time of melanoma and thyroid cancers suggests that these cancers may be more sensitive to the effects of high-frequency transients than the other cancers seen in this population. Of interest, malignant melanoma and thyroid cancer are amongst the highest rates of increase in Western populations.[5]

Milham has been following some of the teachers and students of the La Quinta Middle School since the cancer cluster determination. In April 2008, three former students in their mid-twenties had been diagnosed with thyroid cancer and another had died of breast cancer. Also, a 30-year-old woman had two primary invasive malignant melanomas and in 2009 had both breasts removed (one prophylatically) for breast cancer in one breast. A second teacher in their group also had a case of PCV, in addition to the Burkitt's lymphoma that killed him. Milham reports there were two cases of PCV in the population of these teachers – about 60 times what would be expected.

As Milham and Morgan reported that magnetic fields showed no association, how could dirty electricity create conditions to allow cancer to develop? Milham and Morgan postulated that the dirty electricity in the classroom wiring induced electrical currents in the teachers' bodies. To explain this further, in addition to being part of an electrical circuit because of the electrical Earth currents, each person is part of the transfer of energy within an electrical network to the wires running around them through the walls, floors and ceiling of the building where they work or live.

Our health, strength and endurance depend upon the energy currents that run throughout the body, which exert their effect by capacitive coupling.

Both leukemia and brain tumors feature prominently in the growing cancer story in regard to dirty electricity. The study also focused attention on Elgin-Millville High School in Minnesota where a teacher who had taught in a room that had high levels of dirty electricity died of brain tumors. Another teacher in an adjoining room died of leukemia. Teachers are studied as they are normally exposed to similar working environments. The pattern of cancer increase at La Quinta Middle School is also identical to that found in a large study of cancer incidence in California Teachers Association members in the late 1990s.[6]

Milham and Morgan reported that magnetic fields showed no association with cancer incidence in this study. By delving deeper into how dirty electricity is created and how it can play a role in cancer and disease states, the culprits can be found in our everyday use of electrical equipment and electronics.

Hazelwood School, Australia – Cancer Cluster

Outcome of the official investigation

In late February 2009, an investigation began into the electromagnetic environment at Hazelwood School, Moonah, Tasmania. The school is close to transmission lines supplying power to a zinc smelter and has an electrical substation in the basement. There was excessive corrosion in the water pipes which suggested electrical ground currents in the water system. Most significantly, the swimming pool had to be closed and drained because people were getting electrical shocks when entering the water.

The Department of Health and Community Services conducted a survey wherein detailed EMR measurements were carried out using new equipment, to give a better idea of exposures in multiple locations in classrooms and offices over a period of time. EMR levels were reported as low. The Public and Environmental Health Service also looked for causal factors and environmental hazards.

Tasmanian EMR consultant Don Maisch of EMFACTS Consultancy offered his services free of charge. He had been watching this investigation closely and comments that the survey was conducted only *after* extensive electrical work was carried out at the school to rectify a major ground-current leakage problem that would have resulted in excessive magnetic fields in the building.

According to a staff member – as reported by Don Maisch – about two weeks prior to this survey, the Department of Education had extensive electrical work carried out at the school, including replacement of circuit boards. Maisch comments that it is interesting that the mitigation work was carried out just at the time the department was concerned that a former staff member was considering taking legal action.

Cancers among staff included breast (eight cases), colon, lung, skin, cervical and haemopoietic cancers (including lymphomas). These are cancers that feature quite prominently in environments with high levels of dirty electricity.

Maisch reports that the students were not studied, in part because as a group they have a range of serious conditions. Some of their genetic conditions are already associated with a high risk of cancers, including leukemia early in life.

If EMR exposure is capable of exacerbating their pre-disposition, surely more could be done on a preventative level to ensure they are in a clean electrical/electromagnetic environment.

Chicks after 30 minutes of dirty electricity exposure

In an experiment conducted by Dave Stetzer and Martin Graham, and repeated by professor Yuri Grigoriev, baby chicks were hatched in an incubator. In this photo from Experiment No.2 by professor Yuri Grigoriev (Moscow, March 29, 2004), the chick on the right was not exposed to dirty electricity. The chick on the left is an example of what the chicks looked like after the eggs were exposed to dirty electricity for 30 minutes on the tenth day. A deformed foot and burn like marks were visible.

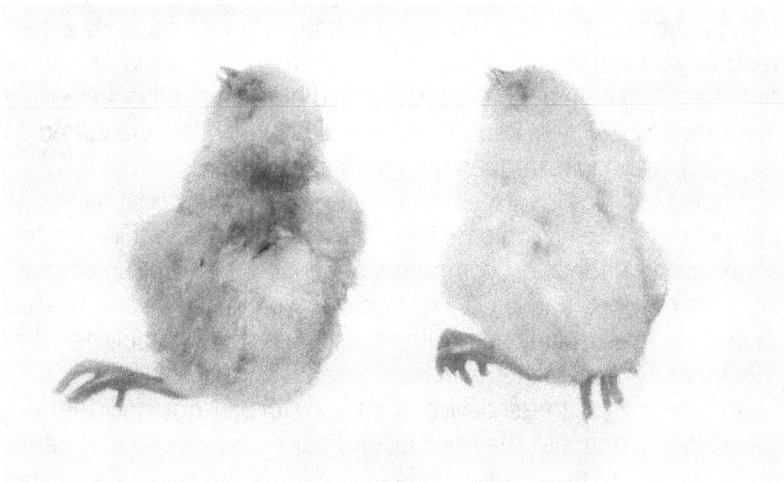

04

THE MISSING LINK

'Dirty electricity is adversely affecting the lives of millions of people.'

Dr Magda Havas and **Dave Stetzer** – presenting at WHO conference

USA 'poor power' quality expert, Dave Stetzer, has researched dirty electricity for decades. Due to his top-secret military clearance in the US Air Force, where he diagnosed, maintained and repaired highly classified crypto electronic equipment, he was cautiously screened by Russian authorities before he was permitted to conduct further studies with the leading specialists from Russia and the Republic of Kazakhstan. Combined with research from the Ukraine, their pooled research confirmed a frequency range that is 'biologically active' – those frequencies can have an effect on living organisms, good or bad or even neutral effects that are neither good nor bad but perceived in some way by the organism. In 2003 the Republic of Kazakhstan swiftly mandated to address the 1 kHz – 400 kHz frequency to protect its citizens.

Why dirty electricity is such a menace is that virtually all of today's energy-efficient equipment and electronic devices draw their needs within this frequency range: most laptops and computers generate 12.5–25 kHz, printers, photocopiers, PlayStations and most electronic equipment generate 10–100 kHz. These fields are particularly harmful because it has been established that this electromagnetic energy penetrates the human body at 1.7 kHz.

Of importance is that these devices create distortion not only inside a building's electrical system, but they also disturb our body's electrical systems.

When exposed to dirty electricity, the electrons in the body are excited and start to oscillate at the same rate as the dirty electricity. This causes internal fields that can damage cells and the induced currents disturb vital intercellular communications.[1]

Computers and children

Dr Vladimir Kozlovsky, highly respected professor of Medicine and Science and deputy director BSE of Infracos-Ecos, Almaty, Kazakhstan, compiled a list of norms that need to be in place to limit children's exposure to computers based on their age.[2] He suggested that:

- children under seven years be exposed for no more than five minutes
- primary school children be exposed for no more than ten minutes
- fifth grade and older children be limited to 30 minutes per day
- teenagers older than 16 years limit their computer exposure to less than three hours daily
- pregnant women should not be exposed to computers at all.[3]

The increasing use of computers and other electrical devices creates this current, which is considered harmful. The wiring in our buildings act as antennae for the current, silently assaulting those who work, live and sleep in the buildings. The wires that deliver electricity everywhere have effectively become a conduit for this harmful energy. We are surrounded by these fields, which now exist potentially on all electrical wiring. Bursts of electromagnetic radiation pack a big burst of energy into a short period of time. For example, a plasma TV sends harmful energy outwards which is absorbed by the body.

High measurements of magnetic fields have long been a concern with all things electrical, but normally the measurements drop off quickly from the source. However, these transient EMF can extend further, and when people are surrounded by other electrical equipment within the room this field is even more concentrated.

Culprits include:

- televisions
- printers
- computers
- power tools
- photocopiers
- fax machines
- dimmer switches
- fluorescent lighting
- medical equipment
- entertainment units
- variable-speed motors
- energy-efficient lighting
- energy-efficient appliances

- power lines that are loose or in contact with trees
- mobile phone masts, broadcast masts (if not properly filtered)

Measuring dirty electricity

As the scientists in the Republic of Kazakhstan understood, there is an urgent need for all people to measure for dirty electricity in their homes and workplaces. Martin Graham, emeritus professor of Electrical Engineering and Computer Science at the University of California, Berkeley, USA, due to his genius, was approached to design a meter to measure the actual amount of this harmful electrical pollution.

The STETZERiZER microsurge meter measures the energy associated with dirty electricity in GS (Graham Stetzer) units with a range up to 1999 GS units. Any measurement over 1999 GS units – over the scale – displays the numeral '1' on the screen. The number on the meter matches the waveform from the oscilloscope.

Everyone can simply plug this meter into an electrical socket in the wall to find what levels of dirty electricity are in their personal environment. The information that an oscilloscope graph shows is now simply represented by a number on the STETZERiZER meter in real time.

GS units, is a new term in the electrical world, named in reverence to the co-creators (Martin Graham and Dave Stetzer) of the STETZERiZER system, who persistently worked on this serious public health issue which medical legal experts consider will dwarf the cigarette smoking and asbestos issues combined. Even though dirty electricity is such a serious threat to our health, this meter is easy to understand:

- 50 GS units is roughly 2 kHz
- The meter measures 1 kHz–150 kHz
- This energy enters the body at roughly 1.7 kHz
- Ensure you are in an environment where it measures under 30 GS units to prevent your body absorbing this radio frequency energy

The measurement of a magnetic field is termed in milliGauss (mG) units, named after Carl Gauss. He also has the Gaussmeter named after him. Nikola Tesla has the microTesla/nanoTesla unit named after him, as some countries use this term instead of milliGauss in his honor. The challenge of devising the STETZERiZER meter has now been respected and Martin Graham and Dave Stetzer's ground-breaking work will be honored throughout history.

Higher cancer incidences in schools and workplaces are more obvious as, apart from the higher concentration of people in these buildings, dirty electricity has been found to be especially prevalent in environments with concentrated fluorescent lights and computers. Milham and Morgan used the STETZERiZER microsurge meter (referred to as the GS microsurge meter in the study) for the La Quinta Middle School study. Twenty-five percent of all rooms at this school measured over the scale.

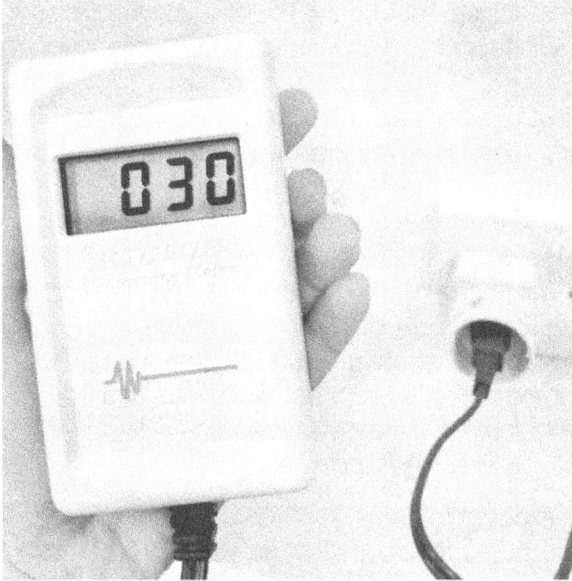

The STETZERiZER Meter displays 30 GS units.

The use of this meter in the cancer cluster at La Quinta Middle School brought further validation on the dangers of exposure to dirty electricity, providing critical information that must be incorporated into our daily lives.

What is important is that dirty electricity showed a positive correlation to cancer incidence at this school:

- Exposure of 1000 GS unit-years increased a teacher's cancer risk by 13%
- Working in a room with a GS overload of more than 2000 GS units for one year increased a teacher's cancer risk by 26 percent

    (To put 26 percent into perspective, those with the BRCA1 and BRCA2 susceptibility genes are considered to be in the highest risk category for breast cancer. In women, mutations in these genes confer a 40-70 percent risk of breast cancer over the course of their lives. Twenty-six percent over one year is therefore extremely high, even without the addition of further years.)

- A single year of employment at this school increased a teacher's cancer risk by 21 percent.

With the teachers being exposed to such high GS units, when no more than 30 GS units are recommended, emphasizes the importance of cleaning up our electrical environments. There is no safe level of exposure.

Graham and Stetzer have provided a solution with the STETZERiZER filters. The compact STETZERiZER (GS) filters were designed to remove this harmful electrical pollution. The filters capture the undesirable high frequencies and transients on the wiring shorting them out, cleaning up the sine wave (signal) or power.

The Republic of Kazakhstan's mandate of 50 GS units addresses the 1 kHz – 400 kHz frequency. The filters are designed from approximately 1 kHz – 400 kHz, with optimum filtering capacity between 4 kHz and 150 kHz. This is the frequency range that weapons experts have identified should be protected. Placed into the power sockets, the appropriate number of filters in a home or building will remove the dirty electricity. The filters do not remove the much higher frequencies of wireless communications.

Why researchers went to such desperate measures to have the La Quinta Middle School cancer cluster examined – which has worldwide ramifications for all of us – is that Milham found if you are exposed to dirty electricity for 6 hours for 180 days a year, your cancer risk is increased by:

- 25 percent if you are exposed to above 2000 GS units
- 15 percent if you are exposed to above 1000 GS units

The increased prevalence of this radiofrequency (RF) current has coincided with an alarming increase in the following health disorders:

- asthma
- ADD and ADHD
- multiple sclerosis (MS)
- CFS
- fibromyalgia

In regard to ADD and ADHD, Milham comments that dirty electricity 'hypes them up'. Milham notes that in the 1973 book, *Health and Light*, John N Ott described a 1973 study of four first-grade classrooms in a windowless Sarasota, Florida school. Two of the rooms had standard white fluorescent lighting and the other two had full-spectrum fluorescent lighting, with a grounded aluminium wire screen to remove the RF radiation produced by fluorescent bulbs and ballasts. Concealed time-lapse cameras recorded student behavior in classrooms for four months. In the unshielded rooms, the first graders developed, '… nervous fatigue, irritability, lapses of attention and hyperactive behavior … students could be observed fidgeting to an extreme degree, leaping from their seats, flailing their arms and paying little attention to their teachers.' In the RF-shielded rooms, 'behavior was entirely different. Youngsters were calmer and far more interested in their work.'

Milham notes Stetzer states dozens of cases of childhood ADHD have been 'cured' with no further need for drugs by simply changing their electrical environments.

Canadian study

Havas is one of the leading experts in dirty electricity research and her studies with Stetzer are increasingly reporting that dirty electricity is: interfering with education in schools and contributing to behavioral problems among students,[4] exacerbating symptoms for those suffering from tinnitus and MS, and contributing to EHS, the most widely reported symptoms being fatigue and mental impairment (poor memory, reduced concentration, and lowered clarity of thought). Complaints also include severe headaches, altered sleep patterns, blurred vision, skin rashes and pain.

Results of removing dirty electricity

The use of the STETZERiZER filters has seen dramatic results. Individuals with MS have had their symptoms diminish, reporting better balance and fewer tremors. Those requiring a cane walked unassisted within a few days to weeks after the filters were installed in their home. Dramatic results have been felt only hours after installation. Several individuals with tinnitus, who have tested the installation of STETZERiZER filters, have reported a significant reduction in the volume of the sound they hear. Some have noticed that when the buzzing is loud, the dirty electricity in their home is high.

Fewer and less severe headaches, more energy and less absenteeism are reported in schools that have installed these filters. Improved behavior associated with ADHD in students has also been reported.

The most impressive result in the schools is in regard to students with asthma. After filters were installed in one Wisconsin school, of the 37 students who had previously used inhalers daily, only three required inhalers, and then for exercise-induced asthma only. After another school in the USA installed filters, a lawsuit initiated by the teachers' union was dropped.

Milham comments that eventually the La Quinta Middle School did spend a small fortune to shield room 304 from high magnetic fields. For about $5000 they could have filtered the whole school and removed the dirty electricity hazard.

Spontaneous abortions

Stetzer examined a bank building in his area of Wisconsin and found women bank clerks were having difficulty getting pregnant or were suffering spontaneous abortions. On examining the bank and finding high levels of dirty electricity, STETZERiZER filters were installed to reduce the levels. A year or so later, he received a telephone call from the bank manager stating that many of the women had left simultaneously on maternity leave.

When Milham looked at the history of the electrification of the USA, he noticed that the more electrification that existed, the lower the fertility and birth rates became. In one place, the birth rate dropped within a year of electrification. In another place, the birth rate was lower in women who didn't practice family planning in an electrified village, compared to women who didn't practice family planning in a village without electricity.[5]

After Stetzer filtered a mid-western school in the USA, a dairy farmer a quarter of a mile away noticed that his cows each gave an average 10 pounds more milk per day, beginning the day the school was filtered. The cows were responding to the dirty electricity being removed from the ground currents, as most of the electricity is sent back via the ground and not the neutral wire. The paper 'Dirty Electrical Power Affects Cows' shows that the number of high frequency events correlates closely with milk production – greater numbers of high frequency events correlated with lower milk production and lower numbers of high frequency events correlated with higher milk production.[6]

Stetzer appears as an expert witness in court cases for farmers, as dirty electricity is not only blamed for lowered milk production in cows, but also in their bearing of deformed offspring. Their families also become ill. It is this area that spear-headed Stetzer's research into dirty electricity.

Other specialists researching dirty electricity include:

- Dr Donald Hillman, emeritus professor, Michigan State University, USA
- Dr Magda Havas, associate professor, Trent University, Peterborough, Canada
- Dr Art Hughes PhD, Electrical Engineering, Texas, USA
- Dr Vitaly Resnik PhD, Republic of Kazakhstan
- Dr Yuri Grigoriev PhD, Moscow, Russia
- Dr Nikitina Valentina, Doctor of Medicine, St Petersburg, Russia.

Milham states dirty electricity explains why professional and office workers have higher incidence rates of cancer, why indoor workers have higher malignant melanoma rates and why melanoma in general can occur on parts of the body that are never exposed to sunlight.

The ground-breaking study at La Quinta Middle School, one of the most significant of our times, strongly indicates the need for the mandatory measuring and filtering of all buildings world-wide.

In 2007, the WHO stated, 'acute biological effects have been established for exposure to ELF electric and magnetic fields in the frequency range up to 100 kHz that may have adverse consequences on health. Therefore, exposure limits are needed.' [7]

In 2011, RF EMF (Radio Frequency EMF) was classified as an IARC 2B (possible) carcinogen. Transient EMF generated in the intermediate frequency at the lower end of RF has characteristics of both ELF EMF and RF EMF. Transient EMF, with its own additional characteristics, is a parasite riding along our 50/60 Hz wiring and spiking further into RF EMF, exacerbating the adverse effects associated with ELF EMF and RF EMF.

05

AGING, DIABETES, EHS, CFS, MS

'According to Philips and Philips (2006) 3% of the population has electromagnetic hypersensitivity (EHS) and 35% have symptoms of EHS. If these percentages apply to diabetics then as many as 5–60 million diabetics worldwide may be responding to the poor power quality in their environment.'

Dr Magda Havas – *Electromagnetic Biology and Medicine, 2006*

Aging

In general, clinical exposure from EMF exposure resembles premature aging.[1] Symptoms of Rapid Aging Syndrome (RAS) include: poor sleep, confusion, chronic fatigue, chronic pain, anxiety and depression and a host of other symptoms treated with pharmaceuticals.

In 2001 a study conducted in Spain examined symptoms experienced by people at various distances from a mobile phone base station.[2] According to the study, people who live within 300 metres of mobile phone towers have an increase in these symptoms:

- *fatigue*
- *sleep disturbance*
- headaches
- feeling of discomfort
- *difficulty concentrating*
- *depression*
- *memory loss*
- *visual disruptions*

- irritability
- *hearing disruptions*
- *skin problems*
- *cardiovascular*
- *dizziness*
- *loss of appetite*
- *movement difficulties*
- nausea

Havas states collectively these symptoms are called EHS – Electromagnetic Hypersensitivity. The symptoms in *'italic'* are the ones we experience as we age. Many people who are EHS attribute their symptoms to aging and leading a stressful lifestyle and become accustomed to chronic ill health.

Diabetes

The number of individuals diagnosed as 'diabetic' worldwide has increased dramatically, as these figures show: 1985 – 30 million, 1995 – 135 million, 2000 – 177 million, 2008 – 250 million, 2025 – 300 million (estimated).

The progress of disease is often invisible, yet with diabetes the health effects of dirty electricity can be measured. The STETZERiZER microsurge meter and the STETZERiZER filter show mathematically and scientifically – the hallmark of acceptance – how dirty electricity can alter bodily processes.

For instance, it has been shown that entering an electrically dirty room can raise blood sugar levels and leaving that room can lower blood sugar levels. Millions of people may discover dirty electricity to be the underlying cause of their 'diabetes' and on its removal they are no longer 'diabetic'.

The meter and filter system is a valuable tool to measure mathematically the lowering of the levels when the filter is installed in the power point. For example, if the meter reads 1700 GS units before the filter is installed, it may read only 1300 GS units after installation. More filters placed in appropriate power points around the building can bring that figure down closer to zero.

The following study shows how dirty electricity can be measured *scientifically.* In 2004, Havas and Stetzer presented this model to the WHO:

	WEEK	DIRTY ELECTRICITY	BLOOD SUGAR	
		GS units	mmoles/L	units
With dirty electricity	1	800	9.4	36
With dirty electricity removed	2	13	6.4	9
% Reduction	0	(98%)	(32%)	(75%)

PPG: >7 mmoles/L is considered by the American Diabetes association to be diabetic.

Model: Electrical Pollution Taskforce, Markham, February 2005 – Dr Magda Havas

(Author's note: A recently published study in the Journal of the National Cancer Institute reported that women with higher insulin levels who are overweight had greater odds of developing breast cancer.) [3]

The above model, which shows the difference between an environment with dirty electricity (800 GS units), and one that has been filtered (13 GS units) provides support for two important conclusions: some diabetics may be over-medicating themselves, and some may be diagnosed with diabetes when they are not diabetic at all.

In mid 2008, Havas labeled environmental diabetes 'type 3' diabetes. This refers to a diabetic whose blood sugar level is also affected by an environmental trigger, such as dirty electricity. Havas' studies show that when dirty electricity is reduced in the home of diabetics, symptoms can diminish. Diabetics with EHS have higher plasma-glucose levels and require more medication when exposed to dirty electricity. [4]

Other studies have also shown that in an electrically clean environment: type 1 diabetics require less insulin and type 2 diabetics have lower levels of plasma glucose.

Havas suggests that dirty electricity may explain why brittle diabetics have difficulty regulating blood sugar. Havas reports that all the diabetics living near relay antennas can easily prove the damaging effects of exposure to artificial high frequency microwave radiation by observing the spectacular increase in blood sugar levels when they are close to a source of radiation, as can be seen from the reading noted in their personal glycaemia record. Havas has also shown that radiation from Digital Enhanced Cordless Telecommunications (DECT) phones can cause an instant change in heart rate and rhythm in some exposed individuals.

Milham reports that the major mortality and morbidity in diabetics is due to acceleration of cardiovascular disease and suggests the blood glucose connection could be how dirty electricity increases cardiovascular disease incidence. [5]

Diesel generator sets are a major source of dirty electricity today and are used almost universally to electrify small islands and places unreachable by the conventional electric grid. Milham states this accounts for the fact that diabetes prevalence, fasting plasma, glucose and obesity are highest on small islands and other places electrified by generator sets and lowest in places with low levels of electrification like sub-Saharan Africa and east and southeast Asia.

Electromagnetic Hypersensitivity (EHS)

EHS is a syndrome that is severely debilitating for increasing numbers of the population and those affected respond more severely, with obvious symptoms. Even though many do not feel these invisible and silent EMF they are still affecting sensitive bodily processes.

Dr William Rea, a former surgeon from Texas determined that his allergic and neurological symptoms were caused by the EMF in the operating room. Rae established the Environmental Health Center in Dallas where his patients were tested through exposure to a spectrum of EMF. It was done in such a fashion that they were unaware of the testing, proving that EHS is a real clinical entity.

In 2004, the WHO organized an international seminar and working group meeting in Prague on EMF Hypersensitivity. At that meeting they defined EHS as follows:

> ... a phenomenon where individuals experience adverse health effects while using or being in the vicinity of devices emanating electric, magnetic, or electromagnetic fields (EMFs) ... Whatever its cause, EHS is a real and sometimes a debilitating problem for the affected persons ... Their exposures are generally several orders of magnitude under the limits in internationally accepted standards.

Dr Olle Johansson, a neuroscientist at the famous Karolinksa Institutet in Stockholm estimates 50 percent of the population of the industrialized world will be EHS by 2017.

EHS is recognized as a disability in Sweden – officially, a fully recognized functional impairment – and just recently also in Canada. In the United Kingdom, it is recognized as a 'condition'. EHS is recognized by the United States Access Board, an independent federal agency whose primary mission is accessibility for people with disabilities. In September 2008, the European Parliament recognized the emergence of EHS.

There are protected living areas in Sweden reserved for the EHS. The first European EHS White Zone is located in the southeast of France, with emergency accommodation for those with EHS who need somewhere to recuperate and heal, and chalets for permanent living.

A specially planned refuge zone for EHS sufferers opened in Italy in 2010. Everything in the Italian zone is free, including the bed & breakfast called 'The Wolf's Hideaway'. The building was restored and shielded with anti-EMF insulation, particularly the bedrooms, and it has space for five EHS guests. A Faraday Cage is now available for extreme cases to be used for a short period of time upon arrival.[6]

The Copenhagen Resolution of October 9, 2010 has called for: more White Zones to be established, EHS be officially recognized as a functional impairment, lowering of guideline levels, and official warnings and protection for the general public from wireless microwave radiation.

Chronic Fatigue Syndrome (CFS)

CFS has been found to be widespread in the electronics industry, particularly in IT workers in Silicon Valley. It has also been noted in Japan where CFS and depression are rampant, that younger people are often showing deterioration of mental faculties similar to that of the elderly. The young are withdrawing from society and shutting themselves off in their rooms.

'About 70 percent of the withdrawn Japanese children have CFS with reduced blood flow to the brain,' says professor Teruhisa Miike of Kumamoto University Medical School. His investigation of cerebral blood flow among children failing to attend school showed reduced blood flow in 75 percent of the cases. Miike states that their failure to attend school is not a 'psychological problem' but a serious illness accompanied by disorders in central nervous system function and immune function.

This CFS may be caused by electromagnetic waves according to a study by Ryoichi Ogawa, a physician in Kobe who suggests that, 'reduced cerebral blood flow may possibly result from the influence of electromagnetic waves from IT equipment'. Dr Ogawa noted that about 80 percent of his CFS patients were frequent users on a daily basis of mobile phones, personal computers, TV games and other IT devices.

Exposure that does not lead to immediate symptoms can still result in cumulative damage that can cause serious disease. Next time the health complaints of a person in a workplace are shrugged off be careful that this warning signal is not ignored. Pay attention as it is most probably the dirty electrical environment that is also silently and unknowingly harming everyone in the office.

Multiple Sclerosis (MS)

Havas states: 'The connection between exposure to artificial electromagnetic radiation in high and low frequencies and the changing health of diabetics and MS sufferers is an established fact that has been demonstrated beyond doubt in numerous scientific studies.' [7]

Havas comments that one teacher in the Wisconsin school that was filtered had been diagnosed with MS. She was extremely tired, had double vision, had cognitive difficulties and could not remember the names of the students in her 4th grade class. Her health would improve during the summer, but her symptoms returned in September. She assumed her problems were mold-related but her symptoms did not improve after the mold was removed from the school. Once the school was filtered her symptoms disappeared.[8]

Many of the symptoms of EHS closely resemble the symptoms of MS. The symptoms of EHS, CFS, fibromyalgia and Gulf War Syndrome are all virtually identical to those of RF sickness. EHS people are the 'canaries in the coal mine' who immediately feel the effects of radiowaves. We are all sensitive to electromagnetic radiation though, and every person is affected by electrical poisoning.

Latest Research on EHS

High histamine levels are common in people with EHS. EHS people are most probably under-methylated: if you are under-methylated you can't break down histamine. The book *Nutrient Power: Heal your Biochemistry and Heal your Brain* by William J Walsh PhD gives further information on under-methylation and over-methylation.

06

DIRTY ELECTRICITY AND BREAST CANCER

'A substantial body of scientific evidence indicates that exposures to common chemicals and radiation, alone and in combination, are contributing to the increase in breast cancer incidence observed over the past several decades.'

Janet Gray, Nancy Evans, Brynn Taylor, Jeanne Rizzo, Marisa Walker
– State of the Evidence: The Connection Between Breast Cancer and the Environment, 2010

Twenty-three years after the atomic bombs were dropped in 1945, it was confirmed and quantified in 1968 that the ionizing radiation (gamma rays) released from the bombs can cause breast cancer.[1] It was many years before Western scientists acknowledged that the resulting sickness came from the radiation from the bombs. It took many decades for scientists to understand how this affected our bodies.

The EMF (non-ionizing radiation) breast cancer connection in women has been hotly debated since the first study reporting a connection in the Western world in 1982. The study was initially intended to look at the overall cancer risk in adults, but found accelerated development and growth of breast cancer, particularly among women younger than 55 years.[2] (An increase in excess cancers of the nervous system, uterus, and lymphoid tumors in adults was also indicated).

In 1997, Dr Thomas Erren, Institute and Policlinic for Occupational and Social Medicine, University of Cologne, Germany determined that an ELF EMF-male breast cancer association is supported.[3]

When three cases of male breast cancer showed up in the same small office in Albuquerque in 2001, Milham testified for the men, arguing that the cancers were caused, in part at least, by EMF (approximately 92mG units) from an electrical vault that was next to the basement office where the men worked. Milham at the time was unaware of dirty electricity.

Milham commented in 2006 that, after Gene Matanoski first announced an EMF-male breast cancer link in 1991, there have been 14 additional studies reporting a similar association. In 2010, Milham stated that there have been 15 studies linking male breast cancer with EMF exposure and that it is so unusual and so consistent he would consider *male breast cancer a sentinel cancer for EMF exposure like mesothelioma is a sentinel for asbestos exposure.* A recently published meta-analysis of 18 studies showed a statistically significant association between EMF exposures and breast cancer among men.[4]

There are currently reports of an epidemic of male breast cancer at the Marine Corps Base Camp Lejeune in North Carolina. The Marines had identified 55 male breast cancer cases and thought the epidemic was caused by solvent contamination of drinking water at the base. Milham, whose work is pivotal in this area and whose research is spread throughout this book, comments that while there are studies that link solvents with a few cancers, the more likely culprit is EMF.

For his 2000 childhood leukemia study, Milham discovered by accident some USA statistics that revealed female breast cancer, as far back as 1930, showed an 80 percent correlation with residential electrification. He states he was so 'blown away' he researched further and eventually, with the help of statistics, exposed the dirty electricity plague.

However due to the currently acknowledged breast cancer risks attributed to reproductive factors, it is easier for the EMF association in women to be masked.

The incomplete investigation in Brisbane, Australia of the electrical environment at the Toowong ABC TV studios' breast cancer cluster is explained further in *Silent Fields – The Growing Cancer Cluster When Electricity Kills.* To date, 18 women in one small area of this workplace developed breast cancer.

In November 2008, professor David Roder, head of Research and Information Science at Cancer Council SA (South Australia), released a report into the investigation of the breast cancer cluster in Australia's Adelaide Women's and Children's Hospital. The maternity and neonatal care ward was the area of concern. Humidicribs can have very high levels of EMF. Due to this, those caring for the infants are also exposed to high EMF.

Professor Roder found nine more cases of breast cancer than might normally occur in a workforce of a similar size, yet he concluded that the higher than usual number was a random occurrence and there was no apparent causal environmental agent that could be linked to the elevated number of cases.

Explanations of 'random' and 'coincidence' occur far too frequently in an age where awareness and integrity must be willing partners with science in addressing the growing cancer cluster story. In 2008, the USA alone had 108 known breast cancer clusters and Australia's figure is rising.

In 2008, an article posted at *Microwave News* reported eight women who worked in the literature building at the University of California, San Diego (UCSD), had developed breast cancer between 2000 and 2006.[5]

Cedric Garland, an epidemiologist at UCSD reported that the number of breast cancer cases alone was significantly more than would have been expected by chance. In his report, he noted that the risk of invasive breast cancer for employees in the literature building appeared to be four to five times higher than that of the general Californian population. In his June 2008 report to Marye Anne Fox, UCSD chancellor and a professor of Chemistry, Garland focused on the possible role played by EMF, especially 'transients' from the motors of the building's elevators.

Since the 1970s, there has been an 80 percent rise in breast cancer cases in the United Kingdom.[6] Between 1973 and 1998, breast cancer rates in the United States increased by more than 40 percent.[7] The use of computers – and the accompanying presence of dirty electricity – has also increased dramatically since the 1970s. Research is continuing into the prevalence of different chemicals as another environmental assault, but, as discussed previously, exposure to EMF has been shown to enhance the damage from other toxic agents.

In regard to dirty electricity, as this energy dissipates into the human body at 1.7 kHz, this means that when you are sitting at a computer plugged into the wall you are sitting in a dirty electrical field, as the computer is generally putting out between 12.5–25 kHz, which is within the 'biologically active' range. This is why we need to be in a filtered electrical environment.

What is also of concern is that these invisible and silent fields are constantly travelling through our bodies, and not only when we are sitting at the computer. They are also riding on the wiring through the walls in our workplaces, schools, hospitals and homes. Traditionally breast cancer was a disease almost exclusively of postmenopausal women, but we are now witnessing women in their twenties and thirties being diagnosed. It follows that the younger the female is when exposed to dirty electricity, the greater her risk of developing breast cancer.

Dirty electricity, known as 'dirty power' by the music industry, is a well-known menace, as it can damage sensitive electrical equipment. Singers with microphones at breast level can also be exposed to dirty electricity.

Artificial radiation

Being born with the silent carrier genes does not cause breast cancer: it increases risk. We must address the causes: the environmental assaults that have increased a woman's lifetime risk of breast cancer so dramatically, from 1:22 in the 1940s to 1:7 in 2004 (USA statistics).

Our history has shown that breast tissue is most sensitive to the artificial electromagnetic radiation that we have created, which is known as ionizing radiation. It is known beyond doubt that the dropping of the atomic bombs on Nagasaki and Hiroshima caused a dramatic rise in breast cancer incidence in survivors. The rates of breast cancer were highest among females younger than 20 years. A significant association was also reported regarding the incidence of male breast cancer. Higher incidence rates of leukemia and salivary gland tumors (now indicated for mobile phone use) were also indicated.

It is becoming apparent that we must all be diligently conscious of any form of artificial radiation and women especially should consider the sensitivity of breast tissue.

The following points illustrate the importance of understanding the different types of artificial radiation we are exposed to:

- Ionizing radiation includes gamma rays from nuclear bombs, X-rays, CT scans and mammograms. Apart from nuclear fallout, exposure to this form of radiation is by choice.
- Non-ionizing radiation includes ELF EMF from electrical wiring, Transient EMF and RF EMF from communication and wireless sources. Exposure to this form of radiation is on unsuspecting recipients.

Being exposed to high measurements of ELF EMF, Transient EMF and RF EMF and also the radiation from mammograms, chest X-rays and CT scans could indeed be a potent stimulus for breast cancer growth.

It is not uncommon for a new technology, that is heralded as the best invention of its time, to later be recognized as producing undesirable effects. Artificially created radiation is no exception to this. The use of X-rays (including mammograms), once believed to be harmless, is now monitored. Precautions are now in place when X-rays are taken, for both the patient and the operator. The amount of radiation a woman is exposed to in a mammogram is now drastically reduced: down from an average 2 rads in 1976 to, depending on several factors, 0.2 rads today. There is wide concern over the over-use of mammograms, especially in younger women, as the challenge of mammography is its ability to cause as well as detect breast cancer. Even though breast cancer awareness, screening and better treatment methods are available, breast cancer incidence continues to increase.

Leading opponents of mammograms are Dr John W Gofman PhD, who reported that past exposure to ionizing radiation – primarily medical X-rays – is responsible for approximately 75 percent of the breast cancer problem in the USA, and Dr Samuel Epstein, chairman of the Cancer Prevention Coalition and emeritus professor of Environmental and Occupational Medicine, University of Illinois School of Public Health, Chicago.

A recently published article in the *British Medical Journal,* 'Breast Screening: The Facts – Or Maybe Not' by Peter Gotzsche and colleagues from the Nordic Cochrane Centre, found women are given one-sided information on screening. The article stated that the leaflet women are given doesn't provide adequate information on the risks of screening for mammograms.

Further to this, Dr Michael Baum, emeritus professor of Surgery at University College, London wrote a letter signed by 22 others – representing public health, oncology, GPs, epidemiology and patients – to *The Times* criticizing the information that is given to women who are invited to attend National Health Service (NHS) breast cancer screening.[8] The letter states that women in the UK are not given enough information about the potential harms associated with breast cancer screening and that for every 2,000 women screened, one will benefit (by having her life saved), but 10 will have unnecessary treatment and a further 200 will suffer the worry of being falsely diagnosed with cancer. However, as the letter acknowledges, there is debate about the numbers.

Professor Julietta Patnick, director of the NHS cancer screening programs, countered that this number is closer to an estimated four or five lives saved and four or five women being unnecessarily treated. Dr Paul Pharoah, a Cancer Research UK researcher at the University of Cambridge, said it was 'imperative' that NHS breast-screening leaflets were rewritten. The leaflets are currently undergoing review.

Other concerns are that repeated low-dose exposures over time may have the same harmful effects as a single high-dose exposure, and time of exposure. Medical Tactile Imaging (SureTouch™) is now in various breast clinics within the NHS in the UK and available in other countries. SureTouch™ is being used in conjunction with mammography, ultrasound and MRI technology.

Consequences of radiation ignorance

The progressive Breast Cancer Fund USA reports:

> Research indicates that breast cancer arises for four primary reasons: genetic mutation, altered gene expression, altered cell interaction, or from exposure to agents that alter the body's natural production of estrogen and other hormones.[9]

Recent genetic data indicate that women with some gene mutations (e.g. ATM, TP53 and BRCA1/2) are more likely to develop breast cancer and may be especially susceptible to the cancer-inducing effects of exposures to ionizing radiation (Andrieu, 2006; Berrington de Gonzales, 2009a; Turnbull, 2006).

Use of X-rays to examine the spine, heart, lungs, ribs, shoulders and esophagus also exposes parts of the breast to radiation. X-rays and fluoroscopy of infants irradiate the whole body (Gofman, 1996). Decades of research have confirmed the link between radiation and breast cancer in women, who were irradiated for many different medical conditions, including tuberculosis (MacKenzie, 1965), benign breast disease (Golubicic, 2008; Mattson, 1995), acute postpartum mastitis (Shore, 1986), enlarged thymus (Adams, 2010; Hildreth, 1989), skin hemangiomas (Lundell, 1999), scoliosis (Morin-Doody, 2000), Hodgkin's disease (Bhatia, 2003; Guibout, 2005; Horwich, 2004; Wahner-Roeller, 2004), non-Hodgkin's lymphoma (Tward, 2006) and acne (El-Gamal, 2006). Again, evidence from almost all conditions suggests that exposure to ionizing radiation during childhood and adolescence is particularly dangerous with respect to increased risk for breast cancer later in life.[10]

There is considerable evidence that medical X-rays (including mammography, fluoroscopy and CT scans) are an important and controllable cause of breast cancer (Gofman, 1999; Ma, 2008). Although there has been a significant decrease in exposures to ionizing radiation from individual X-rays over the past several decades, a recent report indicates a sevenfold increase in exposure to medical sources of radiation from the mid-1980s through 2006, primarily arising from the increased use of CT scans and nuclear medicine (NCRP, 2009). In 2007, approximately 72 million CT scans were conducted in the United States (Berrington de Gonzales, 2009b). When a CT scan is directed to the chest, the individual receives the equivalent radiation of 30 to 442 chest X-rays (Redberg, 2009). Recent modeling estimates that use of chest CTs and CT angiography in 2007 alone will lead to an additional 5,300 cases of lung and breast cancer within the next two to three decades (Berrington de Gonzales, 2009b). Other modeling suggests that 1 in 150 women who are 20 years old when they undergo CT angiograms of the chest, and 1 in 270 women (total) having the procedure, will subsequently develop cancers of the chest, including breast cancer (Smith-Bindman, 2009).[11]

Considering the above, we should not be blasé about our exposure to EMF. The Breast Cancer Fund USA supports The BioInitiative Report 2007, a scientific review of over two thousand studies.[12] The report stated that the scientific evidence is sufficient to warrant regulatory action for ELF EMF and is substantial enough to warrant preventative action for RF EMF. Many overlapping exposures occur between ELF EMF, Transient EMF and RF EMF in our daily lives.

Exposure to toxic agents while in the womb is now considered to be a seed for the development of breast cancer later in life. Dr Andrew Goldsworthy, honorary lecturer at Imperial College, London, states:

> The overall conclusion is that the genetic damage from exposure to electromagnetic radiation can have an almost immediate effect on fertility, but damage to the offspring may take several generations to show up. If we do nothing to limit our exposure to electromagnetic radiation, we can anticipate a slow decline in the viability of the human genome for many generations to come. It is ironic that having only just discovered the human genome, we have already set about systematically destroying it.

Other risk factors

Artificial lighting and shift work are contributing factors to ill health, due to their detrimental effect on melatonin levels and the disruption of the natural cycles that govern our bodies. A recent study examined satellite images of 147 communities and compared the co-distribution of Light at Night (LAN) and cancer incidence across these communities. A significant positive relationship was found between intensity of night light and breast cancer, but no such relationship was found between night light intensity and lung cancer.[13]

EMF affect the levels and action of melatonin, thereby giving estrogen an advantage over melatonin – melatonin competes with estrogen for the existing receptor sites. When melatonin levels are low, estrogen levels are high – high levels of estrogen stimulate estrogen-sensitive breast cancer. Night-time melatonin is a relevant anti-cancer signal to human breast cancers and 90 percent of human breast cancers have specific receptors for this signal.[14]

Reduced melatonin production has been linked to not only breast cancer but also prostate cancer. Charles *et al* (2003) report that workers in the highest 10 percent category for EMF exposure were twice as likely to die of prostate cancer as those exposed at lower levels.

Commonalities between breast and prostate cancer suggest similar aetiological risk factors and the involvement of the same causative agents. Pathological abnormalities occur more frequently within the prostate gland than anywhere else in the human male and, like breast cancer, susceptibility genes appear to account for no more than a small proportion of cases.

Preventative strategies

The risk of developing breast cancer is about five times higher in industrialized nations than it is in developing countries that do not have a prevalence of electricity. It is known that breast cancer occurs more frequently in women who live in more affluent areas. A more comfortable lifestyle usually includes computers and more electrical appliances that contribute to dirty electricity.

As the risk of a female developing breast cancer is very high, preventative strategies are necessary. Working long hours at a computer where the environment is not filtered to remove this higher-frequency field is placing one at risk. Dirty electricity is the missing link, giving further understanding to the dramatic increase in breast cancer statistics.

Even though in the last 15 years a decrease in the number of deaths from this disease has been observed in developed countries, there has been an increase in the number of women – and men – being diagnosed with breast cancer worldwide.

Women's breasts are instrumental in the survival of the species and the incredibly high statistics of breast cancer are highlighting the fact that we have 'got it' horribly wrong.

07

RADIO FREQUENCY AND MICROWAVE RADIATION

'If Alice Stewart had discovered that radiation was good for you, she might have won the Nobel Prize, as more than one of her admirers has commented. But since she is the bearer of bad news there's been a tendency to ignore her.'

Gayle Green, *The Woman Who Knew Too Much*, 1999

Health effects related to this area of EMF have been accumulating for decades. In the 1950s and 1960s, workers who built, tested and repaired radar equipment came down with what was later termed 'radiowave sickness', which caused the Russians to study this extensively. During the Cold War, the Russian government was accused of bombarding the United States embassy in Moscow with radio frequency / microwave radiation (RF/MW). The USA instigated the Pandora Project to gather data on the Russian experiment. The American ambassador became ill and was diagnosed with leukemia. His replacement also became ill and was diagnosed with leukemia. Other embassy staff members became ill and had reproductive problems.

In 1976, the genotoxic evidence for radio frequency/microwave radiation was strong enough to be described as 'a well-established fact'. Genotoxic means any substances that damage DNA or chromosomes. A genotoxic substance is mutagenic, carcinogenic and teratogenic. Genotoxic substances can cause cancer, reproductive health effects and neurological damage. In 1976, Russia enacted legislation to ban all microwave ovens in Russia, as they had found that when food was heated in a microwave the cellular information was altered and the vitamin content was depleted. The Russians also decided to adapt a policy of limiting all radio frequency/microwave radiation from broadcast towers.

When official studies showed the Vatican that radiation levels exceeded the levels set by Italian law, the Vatican authorities claimed the site was sovereign territory and therefore they were not obliged to comply, even though medical reports showed that the incidence of childhood leukemia in the two kilometer radius of the Vatican radio site was six times the national average and the rate of tumors in adults was well beyond the norm.

In July 2010, a court-ordered study found that electromagnetic waves beamed by Vatican Radio leave residents living near the station's antennas at a higher risk of cancer. Italy's most prestigious cancer research hospital, Milan's National Tumor Institute, led by Andrea Micheli now admits that there is a connection between radio and microwave radiation and the cancer incidence, supporting the claim of Cesano residents that children living at a distance of 12 kilometers or less from the antennas have a higher chance of dying from leukemia or lymphoma. According to magistrates, the report justifies the current investigation of six officials of Vatican Radio for manslaughter.[1]

There have also been childhood leukemia clusters near powerful (one million watts) military communications transmitters in Hawaii, Guam and Scotland, as were several other clusters near broadcast facilities throughout the world. The Precision Acquisition Vehicle Entry, Phased-Array Warning System – PAVE PAWS – at the US Air Force Base in Barnstable County on Cape Cod, Massachusetts, USA was the focus of several cancer cluster studies, including an elevated rate of rare Ewing's Sarcoma (a malignant tumor often found in bone with a peak occurrence between 10 and 20 years of age). Nantucket Island, off the Cape Cod coast – home to the powerful Loran C Antenna – has significant elevations of total cancers, malignant melanoma, female breast and colon/rectal cancer, and prostate cancer.

Milham predicts the Nantucket Island cancer rates will gradually decline since the Loran C Antenna was turned off in February 2010. Nantucket and Barnstable rank first and second of the 14 Massachusetts counties for all cancers, female breast cancer, colon/rectal cancer, and prostate cancer.[2]

A study based on 92 active air force bases that were in operation during 1950-1969 in the USA reported that nationally, counties with an air force base were found to have significantly higher incidences of cancer mortality during 1950-1989 compared with counties without an air force base. The authors of the study hypothesize that the chronic low intensity microwave exposure to peak pulse patterns – a characteristic of radar – could influence immune competence and account for the high cancer mortality near air bases. They cited a 1979 study by Meecham and Shaw that documents a 20 percent higher mortality rate for residents within two-three miles of the

LA International Airport compared to a neighbourhood eight-nine miles away. In addition to cancers, a higher incidence of birth defects and nervous breakdowns among residents who live near airports was reported in Japan and Great Britain.[3] Since then, airports and air force bases now have many more transmitters and frequencies. Those who work at or near an airport or air force bases are exposed to radar.

Havas stayed at a hotel that was several kilometers away from the Toronto International Airport and was still able to measure the airport radar in her hotel room. Hotel employees had attributed their customer's difficulty sleeping due to air traffic noise. In 1996, Stanislaw Szmiegelski, a researcher in Poland, reported that radar and radio-exposed military personnel had high rates of leukemia and lymphoma.

Dr Robert Davies co-authored a case report showing that police who held radar guns in their laps had about seven times the expected risk of testicular cancer.[4] Some radar equipment operates in the same frequency range as do mobile phones, and other radar systems operate at higher frequencies, around 2000 MHz.

In July 2010, Cordoba researchers reported on exposure to laptops connected to WiFi: sperm mobility decreases and increases in damage to the sperm DNA. This is the first research conducted worldwide on the topic and was presented in October 2010 at the Congress of the American Society for Reproductive Medicine (ASRM) in Denver Colorado, USA.[5]

Dr Neil Cherry contended that all radiation across the non-ionizing electromagnetic spectrum has contributed to the rise in many cancers, particularly breast cancer, brain tumors and leukemia. This part of the electromagnetic spectrum includes RF EMF up to 300 GHz, which wireless technologies utilize.

Any communication device that is not attached to the wall by a wire is emitting radiation. For example:

- the base units of DECT cordless phones are always radiating, even when the phone is not in use. (Cordless analogue-model base units emit radiation only when the phone is active).
- mobile phones that are on but not in use are also radiating. (The mobile is transmitting at maximum power when you connect or disconnect a call, when it is ringing or sending a text message and when it is being switched on)
- mobile phone towers are always radiating
- wireless networks for computers radiate
- wireless microphones to help the hearing-impaired radiate
- wireless baby monitors radiate

RF EMF from wireless technology that flows through the air can be easily received and carried by the electrical wiring network in our buildings. This creates additional dirty electricity and because this electrical wiring network acts continuously as an antenna, our exposure to this radiation is thus increased.

Mobile phone masts and broadcast masts, if not properly filtered, are also a potent source of dirty electricity that is transferred through the electrical grid into surrounding buildings and houses.

International action

In their article Cancer Trends During the 20th Century,[6] Örjan Hallberg and Olle Johansson reported that in the USA, Sweden and dozens of other countries, mortality rates for skin melanoma, bladder, prostate, colon, breast and lung cancers closely paralleled the degree of public exposure to radiowaves during the past one hundred years. When radio broadcasting increased in a given location, so did those forms of cancer, and when it decreased, so did those forms of cancer.[7]

Mobile phone antenna studies are showing that people who live within 400 metres of these antennas experience an increased risk of cancer and symptoms associated with EHS. Associate professor Johansson, along with Brian Stein and Liz Lynne MP, colleagues of Eileen O'Connor of the UK Radiation Research Trust, recently visited residents living in a cancer cluster around a base station in Kingswinford, UK. Fourteen people in this location have died of cancer and a further 20 people in the area have been diagnosed with the disease.[8]

Blake Levitt and Dr Henry Lai in their recent paper report: 'Both anecdotal reports and some epidemiology studies have found headaches, skin rashes, sleep disturbances, depression, decreased libido, increased rates of suicide, concentration problems, dizziness, memory changes, increased risk of cancer, tremors and other neurophysiological effects in populations near base stations.' These symptoms decrease or disappear when the transmitters are turned off (for repair), when people shield their homes from the radiation, or when they leave their immediate environment and are not exposed to this radiation.[9]

The BioInitiative Report 2007 stated that the scientific evidence is substantial enough to warrant preventative action for RF EMF. The report concluded that plausible biological mechanisms had already been identified that can reasonably account for most biological effects of exposure. The BioInitiative Report 2012 called for the adoption of new safety limits for RF EMF.

Since the release of The BioInitiative Report in August 2007, moves to lessen exposure to the explosion of wireless technologies is snowballing. The European Parliament demanded in its resolution of September 4, 2008 that the allowable levels for electromagnetic radiation be considerably reduced with regard to public health.

In December 2008, in Valance, France, both the mayor and the opposition agreed – in a political rarity – to mobile phone masts not being erected within one hundred metres of crèches and schools.

Giving legal recognition to the risks posed to human health by mobile phone masts, a legal precedent was established when the Versailles Court of Appeal ordered the dismantling of an antenna mast in Tassin la Demi-Lune in the Rhone. All relay antennae of that particular telecommunications company were placed under suspended sentence. A September 2008 judgment stated:

> To expose one's neighbour against his will to a certain risk, and not a hypothetical one as the defence has claimed, constitutes in itself a public nuisance. Its egregious character is due to the fact that it has a bearing on human health. If this risk were to materialise in significant health problems, this would constitute a different type of offence deserving a more severe sentence, in accordance with the gravity of the problems.[10]

In March 2009, a judge in Angers Tribunal de Grande Instance (District Court) prevented the Orange phone company installing a mobile phone antenna in the bell tower of a church next to a school.

In February 2009, the Tribunal de Grande Instance (District Court) of Carpentras ordered, on the grounds of potential health risks and nuisance to one's neighbour, the demolition of a relay telephone mast, with a penalty of 400 euros per day of delay after the fourth month of the announcement of the judgement.[11]

In November 2008, Liechtenstein became the first country to mandate lower emission standards – by 10 times – to go into effect in 2013. The emissions from outdoor antennae used by mobile phones, radar, TV and FM broadcasting, and wireless internet are to be 0.1µW/cm² or 0.614 V/m, which is the limit for the city of Salzburg.

Of immense importance, in April 2009, the European Parliament passed the European Parliament EMF Resolution: *Health Concerns Associated with Electromagnetic Fields.*[12]

The Breast Cancer Fund USA states that based on the scientific evidence set forth in The BioInitiative Report and a growing body of additional research, exposure limits for electromagnetic radiation should be set at the federal level. The European Environmental Agency also supported The BioInitiative Report.

Arthur Firstenberg reported in *The Largest Biological Experiment Ever* that two minutes on a mobile phone disrupts the BBB, two hours on a mobile phone causes permanent brain damage and second-hand radiation may be almost as bad.[13]

Mobile phones

In 1974, United States Army researchers reported that low-level microwave radiation – such as that used by mobile phones – might alter the functioning of the blood-brain barrier (BBB). Swedish scientists repeated this warning in 1992 and also suggested a potential link with Alzheimer's and other neurological diseases.

Professor Leif Salford of the Department of Neurosurgery from Lund University in Sweden, who has been researching for over 20 years, has publicly warned that a whole generation of teenagers using mobile phones may suffer from mental deficiencies or Alzheimer's disease by the time they reach middle age.

Johansson reports that when second-generation 1800-MHz mobile phones were introduced into Sweden in 1997, a significant and permanent worsening of the public health began precisely at that time. After a decade-long decline, the number of Swedish workers on sick leave began to rise in late 1997 and more than doubled during the next five years.

During the same period, sales of antidepressant drugs also doubled. The number of traffic accidents, after declining for years began to climb again in 1997. The number of deaths from Alzheimer's disease, after declining for several years, rose sharply in 1999 and had nearly doubled by 2001.[14]

Salford has shown mobile phone radiation results in leakage of the BBB, the biological barrier surrounding the brain which blocks the entry of certain, and possibly harmful, molecules in the general blood circulation from entering the central nervous system. Heavy metals in the brain act as micro-antennae concentrating EMF radiation into the brain. Dental amalgams also increase reception. One of many potential outcomes of BBB leakage is dementia.

When you make a call with a mobile phone, a radio signal travels to the closest base station antenna. The signal is sent from the antenna to the phone you are calling. This radio signal is sent by way of radio frequencies. The antenna inside the mobile phone gives off radio frequencies and some of these are transferred to and absorbed into the head when you are using the phone. The closer the antenna is to your head or body the greater the exposure to RF energy.

When talking on the mobile phone while moving in a car, train or bus, the exposure levels are much higher because of the ongoing reconnection as the vehicle moves forward and also because of the internal reflections in metal vehicles. Airline crew are constantly being exposed to wireless technology in aircraft.

Exposure to RF is greater if you use the mobile phone for long calls or if the closest antenna is far away. Using a mobile phone in rural areas places you more at risk, as rural users are further away from the mobile phone towers compared to urban users, and the mobile phone's radiated power is higher.

The SAR (Specific Absorption Rate) is now given more publicity by the telecommunications companies and supported by federal governments as protecting the public. SAR only regulates against thermal damage – heating – and not the cancer causing effects (non-thermal – biological). It does not indicate whether your phone is 'safe'. The late Dr Robert C Kane, author of *Cellular Telephone Russian Roulette: A Historical and Scientific Perspective*, states that what emerges from the science is clear: both thermal and non-thermal radio frequency radiation can cause brain tissue damage.

In 2013 Belgium banned the sale of mobile phones to children and in 2014 it was announced all mobile phones will be labelled with the letter 'A', 'B', 'C', 'D', or 'E', corresponding to the phone's SAR. 'A' 'indicates a SAR less than 0.4 watts/kilogram (w/kg), 'B' from 0.4 to less than 0.8 w/kg, 'C' from 0.8 to less than 1.2 w/kg, 'D' from 1.2 to less than 1.6 w/kg, and 'E' more than 1.6 w/kg. Phones sold in other countries are measured in a different manner than in European countries.

In 1994, Dr Henry Lai and Dr Narendrah Singh, biomedical researchers at the University of Washington in Seattle, made known the results of their research that should have been received by the mobile phone industry as the conclusive proof it claims to be seeking. Their findings provided a significant confirmation of the previous studies out of India, Belgium and Kiev that reported: low-level radio frequency radiation exposure causes DNA modification.

Lai and Singh repeated the experiments and, in 1996, reported again that low-level exposure to radio frequency radiation causes an increase in single and double-strand breaks in DNA. Lai and Singh, Sarkar, Maes, Cleary and Verschaeve independently found chromosomal and DNA damage as a result of their experiments. Lai summed up the findings by stating:

> DNA damage is related to the initiation of cancer – if there is an error in the repair process, it could lead to a problem. The problem Lai suggests is cancer.[15]

The largest epidemiological investigation ever conducted into the link between cancer and mobile phones – the Interphone studies – were largely funded by the wireless communications industry. Based on data from 13 countries, the Interphone studies concluded that mobile phone exposure did not increase the risk of brain tumors.

In addition to possible bias associated with industry funding, the studies had some important flaws, including relatively short durations of mobile phone use.[16] Also, an independent series of studies led by highly respected Dr Lennart Hardell, a cancer specialist reached a different conclusion.

Hardell's studies included more patients who had used a mobile phone for 10 years or longer and were performed without financial support from the wireless industry. The findings suggested that the more hours of mobile phone use over time, the higher the risk of developing brain tumors. Risk also increased along with the level of power from the wireless device, years since first use, total exposure, and younger age when starting wireless phone use. Generally the studies are finding a statistically increased risk after a 10-year latency period. This is quite rapid for brain tumors, that normally have a latency period of 20 to 30 years in adults.

A study published in the *International Journal of Oncology* was based on the analysis of 1600 tumor victims who had used mobile phones for up to 10 years. Professor Kjell Mild, the Swedish biophysicist who led the study stated: 'The evidence for a connection between phone use and cancer is clear and convincing. The more you use phones and the greater the number of years you have them, the greater the risk of brain tumors.' An earlier study by Mild and Hardell linked brain tumors to analogue mobile phone use. The new research repeated this and also looked at digital mobiles and DECT cordless phones, showing that all three types were linked with increased tumor rates.

In September 2013, Hardell, Mild, Carlberg and Söderqvist stated their findings support the hypothesis that RF EMF play a role in both the initiation and promotion stages of carcinogenesis.[17]

In 2013, Hardell and Carlberg stated, based on the Hill criteria, glioma and acoustic neuroma should be considered to be caused by RF EMF emissions from wireless phones and regarded as carcinogenic to humans, classifying it as group 1 according to the IARC classification. Current guidelines for exposure need to be urgently revised.[18]

Overall, findings from Israel and Sweden indicate a link between long term mobile phone use and three types of tumors: glioma (brain cancer in the brain's glial cells), parotid gland tumor, and acoustic neuroma (a tumor of the auditory nerve in the brain).

Goldsworthy comments:

Heavy mobile phone use appears to reduce both the quantity and viability of sperm. The results for the most recent study by Dr Ashok Agarwal and co-workers at the Cleveland Lerner College of Medicine can be seen at http://tinyurl.com/28rm6n. They found that using a mobile phone for more than four hours a day was associated with a reduction in sperm viability and mobility of around 25 percent. The statistical probability of these results being due to chance errors was one in a thousand. There is every reason to believe that human eggs may be similarly affected, but since they are formed in the embryo before the baby is born, the damage will be done during pregnancy but will not become apparent until the child reaches puberty.

Mobile phones and breast cancer

A study in 2013 reported four young women – aged 21 to 39 – with multifocal invasive breast cancer. They regularly carried their smartphones directly against their breasts in brassieres for up to 10 hours a day for several years and developed tumors in areas of their breasts immediately underlying the phones. They had no family history of breast cancer, tested negative for BRCA1 and BRCA2, and had no other known breast cancer risks. The pathology of all four cases showed striking similarity: all tumors were hormone-positive, low-intermediate grade, having an extensive intraductal component, and all tumors had near identical morphology.[19]

Child protection in Russia

The following report on the dangers of children using mobile phones comes from the Russian National Committee on Non-Ionizing Radiation Protection, Moscow, Russia the most progressive radiation board in the world:[20]

> For the first time in history, we face a situation where most children and teenagers in the world are continuously exposed to the potentially adverse effects of electromagnetic fields (EMF) from mobile phones.
>
> An electromagnetic field is an important biotropic factor, affecting not just human health in general but also the processes of the higher nervous activity, including behavior and thinking. Radiation directly affects the human brain when people use mobile phones.
>
> Despite the recommendations listed in the Sanitary Rules of the Ministry of Health, which insist that persons under 18 years should not use mobile phones, children and teenagers became the target group for the marketing of mobile communications.
>
> The current safety standards for exposure to microwaves from mobile phones have been developed for adults and don't consider the characteristic features of children's organisms. The WHO considers the protection of children's health from the possible negative influence of EMF from mobile phones as the highest priority. This problem has also been confirmed by the Scientific Committee of the European Commission, by national authorities of European and Asian countries, and by participants of international scientific conferences on biological effects of the EMF.
>
> The potential risk for children's health is very high:
>
> * The absorption of electromagnetic energy in a child's head is considerably higher than in an adult's head (children's brains are smaller, have higher conductivity, thinner skull bones, and a smaller distance from the antenna).

- Children's organisms have greater sensitivity to EMF than adults'.

- Children's brains have greater sensitivity to the accumulated adverse effects relating to chronic exposure to EMF.

- EMF affects the formation of the process of the higher nervous activity.

- Today's children will spend significantly more time using mobile phones than will today's adults.

According to the opinion of the Russian National Committee on Non-Ionizing Radiation Protection, the following health hazards are likely to be faced by children using mobile phones in the immediate future: disruption of memory, decline of attention, diminishing learning and cognitive abilities, increased irritability, sleep problems, increase in sensitivity to stress, increased epileptic readiness.

Expected (possible) remote health risks: brain tumors, tumors of acoustical and vestibular nerves (in the age 25–30 age group), Alzheimer's, 'got dementia', depressive syndrome, and other types of degeneration of the nervous structures of the brain (in the 50–60 age group).

The members of the Russian National Committee on Non-Ionizing Radiation Protection emphasize the urgency of defending children's health from the influence of EMF from mobile communication systems. We appeal to government authorities and to the entire society to pay closest attention to this coming threat and to take adequate measures to prevent negative consequences to future generations' health.

Children using mobile communications are not aware of the risks in subjecting their brains to EMF radiation. We believe that this risk is not much lower than the risk to children's health from tobacco or alcohol. It is our professional obligation not to allow this damage children's health by inactivity.

April 14, 2008

Biophysicist Marko Markov PhD, president of Research International in Williamsville, New York USA and Yuri G Grigoriev PhD, chairman of the Russian National Committee on Non-Ionising Radiation Protection, member of the Russian Academy of Electrical Engineering Sciences, the International Advisory Committee of WHO's International EMF Project and the Institute of Electrical and Electronics Engineers in their article, *Wi-Fi Technology an Uncontrolled Experiment on the Health of Mankind,* state this is the first time in the history of our civilization that the most critical systems in the human organism – the brain and the nerve structures inside the internal ear of children and adults – are exposed to complicated and unknown levels of EMF.

They further state:

> Another critical point of consideration is that the energy absorption characteristics that make the 750 and 915 MHz frequencies so desirable for hyperthermia and diathermy treatments have the very same absorption characteristics that make the 825 to 845 MHz cellular telephone transmission band so dangerous (Kane 2001).

> For 825-845 MHz, the penetration depth into the brain tissue is from 2.0 to 3.8 centimetres (Polk & Postow, 1986) ... A number of studies pointed out that electromagnetic energy in the 900 MHz region may be more harmful because of its greater penetrating capability compared to 2450 MHz, therefore, more energy in the 900 MHz frequency range is deposited deeply within the biological tissue. In 1976 Lin concluded that 918 MHz energy constitutes a greater health hazard to the human brain than does 2450 MHz energy for a similar incident power density (Li 1976).[21]

Following on from Israel, in 2015 legislation in France stipulates no wireless devices will be allowed in facilities that cater to children under three years of age and WiFi in schools must be turned off when not being used for educational activities. Israel limits wireless to 1 hour a day in grades 1 and 2, and schools in many countries are now removing WiFi.

Cordless 'landline' phones

Do DECT cordless phones and wireless WiFi routers affect the heart? Havas states:

> Yes. The heart, along with the brain, is an electrical organ, so should we be surprised that these artificial fields that we have created interfere with their function?

> The older analogue cordless phones emitted radio frequency radiation only when you held the phone. The phone bases of the newer DECT phones that operate within frequencies of 1.9 GHz, 2.45 GHz, and even 5.8 GHz, constantly radiate even when you are not using the phone. If you sit or lie near the phone base, you are exposed to unnecessary amounts of RF radiation.

> Cordless phones, whose base stations radiate in an 'always on' mode using 2.4 GHz or 1.8 GHz DECT technology, should be banned. These phones do not always have the frequencies or 'DECT' written on the phone. According to The BioInitiative Report, use of cordless phones predominantly on the same side of the head for more than 10 years increases people's risk of a malignant glioma (brain tumor) by 470 percent.

There is unequivocal evidence that effects have been observed by DECT phones. Havas now, for the first time, has conclusive evidence that this radiation can affect the heart.[22] Symptoms included: palpitations, arrhythmias, pain or pressure in the chest, lowered or heightened blood pressure, and shortness of breath or anxiety.

Using live-blood analysis, I experimented with a DECT phone – 2.4 GHz frequency and 3mW/cm² – for three-minute intervals and two feet from the head. Healthy cells have the cells round and separate, with few sticking together. The electrical charge on the outside of the red blood cells was altered, the cells sticking together like stacked coins after 10 minutes on the cordless phone. There were no single cells and most of the cells were like stacked coins. This type of clumping interferes with the release of oxygen and the removal of waste products like carbon dioxide, resulting in poor circulation. Havas states Live Blood Analysis may be a good diagnosis for those who are EHS.

Because DECT phones are so powerful and because the radiation can penetrate through walls, people in apartment blocks can be exposed to this radiation from a neighboring apartment even if they do not own a DECT phone. Scientists state the damage is caused by the disruption of microtubular connections that allow biophotons to communicate between cells, which decrease intracellular communication. Increased deposits of heavy metals also begin to accumulate in the cells, which increases intracellular production of free radicals and can radically decrease cellular production of energy, thus making people incredibly fatigued.

To check as to whether a cordless phone is analogue or digital, take a portable radio and turn it to an AM station at the lower end of the AM dial and then turn it slightly off station so static can be heard. Bring the radio close to the base station of the cordless phone when it is plugged into an outlet. If louder static can be heard and if this goes away when the cordless phone is unplugged or the radio is moved away from the cradle, the phone is DECT – 2.4 GHz or 1.8 GHz – always on. WiFi uses the same frequencies (2.4 GHz).

In December 2009, the Highest Regional Court in Brescia (North Italy) ruled that INAIL (Istituto Nazionale by l'Assicurazione contro gli Infortuni sul Lavoro, the National Public Insurance Institute) is liable for the brain tumor of an employee. The employee was required to use a mobile phone and cordless phone for many hours each day. As a result of the case, the plaintiff receives an 80 percent disability pension.

This judicial decision makes it possible for Italian employees to insist on using corded phones and advise their employers that they are liable for health effects caused by cordless phones.[23] The German Federal Radiation Protection Agency advises their citizens not to use DECT phones.[24]

Legal precedent

Gloria Vogel, managing director of New York-based Vogel Capital Management, comments that legal precedent has been established in the case of *AT&T Alascom and Ward North America Inc. vs John Orchitt, State of Alaska, Department of Labor and Workforce Development, Division of Workers' Compensation*. The July 2007 ruling affirmed a 100 percent disability award to a worker exposed to RF radiation that only slightly exceeded the FCC human exposure limits. Vogel says that the Alaska Supreme Court established a legal precedent that recognizes the causal link between RF radiation exposure and cognitive or psychological injuries, including reduced brain function, memory loss, sleep disorders, mood disorders and depression.[25]

Wireless smart meters

Wireless 'smart meters' will require a new blanket of wireless radiation over entire communities. Smart meters use radio frequencies to send information about electricity use back to headquarters.

A wireless smart meter produces RF/MW radiation with two antennas in approximately the same frequency range (900 MHz to 2.4 GHz) as a mobile phone tower. Depending on how close it is to occupied space within a home, a smart meter can cause higher RF exposures than towers. Relatively potent and very short pulsed RF/MWs, these milli-second long RF burst on average 9,600 times a day with a maximum of 190,000 daily transmissions.

Stetzer states that the two frequency issues are the transmitted frequency that is transmitting the data through space and the frequency that is created by the switch-mode-power supply.

In order for the meter to transmit, it has to have a transmitter inside of it. Since the transmitter can only operate on DC, the AC that is being supplied to the building has to be changed to DC inside the meter socket only for the transmitter circuit. This is accomplished by the use of a switch-mode-power supply. It chops up the AC sine wave, creating high frequencies and harmonic currents to be put back on the wires of the power grid, as well as every wire in the house or building.

Although the frequency may vary, depending on the type of switch-mode-power supply being utilized, the frequencies are usually 50 kHz. This is right in the middle of the most biologically active frequencies when it comes to human health.

Also of concern is when the meter is mounted on the same wall as a bedroom or a room where any occupant spends a lot of time. Multiple meters, mounted for apartment living just outside living areas and in particular, areas where people sleep, are also a concern. Having multiple meters can cause even higher radiation levels. It appears that each meter transmits radiation at different strengths and at different time periods, depending on the distance the signal has to travel, the physical barriers between the meter and the collection point, and the number of meters using the meter as a stepping stone to pass their information along the line to the collection point.

You may ask that the utility replace the smart meter with a regular mechanical hour-watt meter but you may have to pay the additional cost of having someone come out to manually read your meter. Some countries are making these smart meters mandatory. Milham suggests the billing information could be sent over existing phone lines or fiber optic lines.

According to the USA Department of Energy's October 2010 broadband report on data privacy, 'consumers should have rights to protect the privacy of their own Consumer-Specific Energy Usage Data and control access to it. Well-designed implementations of Smart Grid technologies should also empower individual consumers to make a wide array of choices about whether or how to manage their own energy-consumption data via home energy management systems.' Activists can use this information to demand an opt-out option if a ban on smart meters is not feasible. Many individuals and towns across the world are fighting the installation of smart meters.

In July 2013, a class action lawsuit was filed in the Supreme Court of British Columbia against BC Hydro and Power Authority. It was filed on behalf of everyone in British Columbia who has had a smart meter installed on their houses against their will. The plaintiffs are asking for an injunction ordering the removal of the smart meters, damages for trespass, nuisance, and intrusion against seclusion and punitive damages. Also in 2013 a lawsuit was filed against Southern California Edison and Itron, the company that manufactures the smart meters. The plaintiffs are claiming: negligence, fraud and deceit, intentional infliction of emotional distress and liability for a defective product.

It is understood that by late 2014 Germany has rejected smart meter deployment, and 111 municipalities in Quebec have called for a moratorium and/or free opt out. Italy has also opted for safer, faster and more secure hard-wired technology. Due to fire hazards thousands of smart meters have been removed in Saskatchewan in Canada, and Florida (Lakeland), Pennsylvania and Oregon in the USA.

WiFi and cardiac arrest

Havas comments:

> Whether the issue is WiFi in schools, cell phone use, or living near cell phones antennas ... in all cases people are exposed to microwave radiation. This radiation is similar to what is emitted by microwave ovens. The major difference is

that the radiation in the microwave oven is supposed to be contained, whereas the radiation from all these other devices is not contained. Indeed, it if were contained, the devices would not work.

What happens if you put metal into a microwave oven? It sparks, as it reflects the microwave radiation. The same thing happens in your home. Metal objects reflect this radiation and can produce hotspots.

So, the classroom with the WiFi base station and the bedroom with the cell phone antenna nearby become the microwave ovens with the radiation set on low power.

There is a very disturbing state of affairs being experienced in Ontario Schools. The School Board is threatening to fine parents and to expel students, and they are also threatening teachers who do not toe the line regarding WiFi. What kind of country has Canada become? How can educational authorities be so insensitive, so militant and so ignorant? Perhaps someone should follow the money because none of this makes any sense.

All parents are asking for is that computers be wired when they connect to the internet! In some areas, the parents are even willing to pay for the costs of hardwiring their children's school.

FACT: Students are becoming ill in schools with WiFi.

FACT: Studies are showing that this radiation, at levels well below our guidelines, are making adults sick.

FACT: Parents are trying to protect their children from this radiation and they are going to be fined and their children expelled? For what? For being concerned about a form of radiation that causes cancers, breaks DNA, affects sperm, causes heart irregularities and has been associated with headaches, dizziness, nausea, skin rashes, ringing in the ear.

Today, I learned from a colleague in Switzerland that students in Swiss schools that have WiFi are experiencing the same symptoms that were reported earlier this year in Collingwood.

A few months ago, another colleague told me that during the past year, two students died of cardiac arrest in San Anselmo. One was within 100 meters of a major cell tower and the other was taking a shower at his high school. Instead of putting in defibrillators, shouldn't the school board be asking the question why are there so many heart irregularities among young students and why have at least two students (to my knowledge) in the Collingwood area experienced cardiac arrest within the past year.

Studies show that exercise-related sudden cardiac arrest in youth is on the rise and no one knows why. According to one study (Drezner *et al*, 2008), during a 7-year period (2000-2006) there were 486 cases of sudden cardiac arrest in the US, which comes to an average of 70 cases each year. Based on population size, we might expect 7 cases in all of Canada each year. The number in the Barrie area, within the past year, is much higher than one could expect for such a small population.

The school board is taking the sudden cardiac arrests seriously because they are installing defibrillators to revive students who experience cardiac arrest. That's like issuing epi-pens to students with peanut allergies and encouraging them to eat peanuts!

Where are the health authorities in all of this? Certainly this has received a lot of media attention (TV, radio newspapers), yet I know of no health authorities, local, provincial or federal, who are investigating student ill health and the cardiac problems at these schools. I can't believe that it may take the death of one or more students before we take corrective steps to eliminate whatever is responsible for this health crisis. If it is not WiFi, then let's find out what it is. But, let's not ignore this issue and just hope it will go away, because that is most unlikely.

While school boards in Ontario are planning to expel students who refuse to be exposed to WiFi, in Israel, the Labor, Social Affairs and Health committees are planning to establish cellphone-free zones in schools to minimize exposure of students and teachers to microwave radiation. Israel's Knesset panel endorses minimizing school radiation exposure.

Schools in parts of France, Britain, Canada and elsewhere are quietly replacing WiFi with wired connections. A few school boards in Canada have plans to measure the levels of radiation in the classroom but, I was told, they have no intention of sharing this information with parents or the public! What are they hiding and what are they afraid of? How did we get into this mess in the first place and when will sanity return to the School Trustees and the Health Authorities?[26]

The disappearance of the birds and the bees

In 2008, it was reported that since 2006 beekeepers have documented unexplained losses of hives of 30 percent and upward. According to a USA congressional report, up to 36 percent of 2.4 million bee colonies were wiped out in the 2006/2007 winter – normal winter bee die-off is 10 to 20 percent. USA Congress recognized this phenomenon – colony collapse disorder (CCD) – as a threat and gave the USA Department of Agriculture emergency funds to study honeybee disappearances.

Disappearing bees have also been reported in Europe and Brazil. Canadian beekeepers reported losses of one-third of the country's bees during the 2006/2007 winter, including a 23 percent loss in British Columbia alone. A study, conducted by Jacobus Biesmeijer and William Kunin (Leeds University,

United Kingdom) and a team of British, German and Dutch researchers, and published in *Science*, confirms that the threat is serious. By studying different areas of Great Britain and the Netherlands, scientists observed that wild bees have paid the heaviest toll, with a 52 percent reduction in their diversity with respect to their situation in 1980 in Great Britain and a 67 percent reduction in the Netherlands.

A series of studies have demonstrated the negative effect of pulsed, digital radiation on bees and bee hives.[27] CCD is characterized by the outright disappearance of bees, rather than piles of dead bees in the hives, as would be the case if they died of pesticides, viruses or parasites. Bees have an internal compass containing a mineral called magnetite in their abdomens, which helps them navigate by using the Earth's EMF. Birds also have magnetite in their brains and beaks, which normally helps them with orientation. Are the increasing amounts of electrosmog throwing them off course?

According to Dr George Carlo, who ran the North American wireless industry's 6-year $28.5 million research program, the culprit in the disappearing birds and bees threat is the Information Carrying Radio Waves (ICRW) spread worldwide by mobile phone antennae and other wireless transmissions. Carlo is convinced that the ICRW interfere with intercellular communication in all living things, harming the bees' navigation as well as their immune systems. Carlo believes our environment has reached the saturation point for ICRW.

According to Dr S Vijayan, director of the Salim Ali Centre for Ornithology and Natural History (SACON), 'a number of studies have been conducted to find out the relationship between the increase in electromagnetic waves and the decrease in the number of sparrows. A positive correlation has been found between them. There have been studies in Spain which showed that sparrows disappear from cities where electromagnetic contamination is very heavy.'

In 2014, a study was initiated in London by the British Trust for Ornithology to investigate whether the explosion of electromagnetic waves from portable handsets is wiping out sparrows in London. The British study involves 30,000 birdwatchers, who will examine the urban sparrow population near mobile phone antennas where electromagnetic fields are most concentrated.

London has witnessed a steep fall in its sparrow population – a 75 percent fall since 1994. Vijayan also pointed out that sparrows are found to be disappearing from areas where mobile phone towers are installed. SACON has also initiated a detailed study to find out how exactly these small birds are being affected.

Vijayan stated:

These are all circumstantial evidences. Now we need to prove how it is exactly affecting the sparrows. My feeling is that it probably affects their central nervous system. We are conducting studies with inputs from various cities on the falling number of sparrows in which the effects of electromagnetic contamination from mobile phones are also being examined.

If the decline of the bees continues, it will have a devastating effect on the availability of food for humans. Whatever is causing the decline in bee population in developed countries, it is likely to be artificially produced by humans. Goldsworthy reports various possibilities have been mooted, including the varroa mite, pesticides and other agrichemicals, but the front-runner, for which there is the most convincing evidence, is the RF radiation from mobile telecommunications. Goldsworthy states it looks very much as if it is due to the effects on their cryptochrome pigments.

In reporting that EMF disrupt crypto-chrome-based magnetic navigation, Goldsworthy states it has been shown that even weak electromagnetic radiation, over a wide range of radio frequencies, completely prevented robins orienting for navigation in a steady magnetic field simulating that of the Earth, and the same is probably true for bees.[28] The mechanism has since been confirmed and further elucidated by other workers. The cryptochrome-based body clock in insects is also affected by magnetic fields.[29]

Humans use cryptochromes to control our circadian rhythms and immune systems.

World Cancer Authority — IARC

Only days after the Council of Europe – elders from 47 European countries – called for a dramatic reduction in EMF exposure to humans from wireless technologies, on May 31, 2001 the IARC, the leading cancer authority in the world, classified RF EMF as possibly carcinogenic to humans, based on an increased risk for glioma, a malignant type of brain cancer associated with wireless phone use.

The IARC Monograph Working Group discussed and evaluated the available literature on the following exposure categories involving RF EMF: occupational exposures to radar and to microwaves, environmental exposures associated with transmission of signals for radio, television and wireless telecommunication, and personal exposures associated with the use of wireless telephones.[30]

Alternatives to wireless

Havas comments:

> While the rest of the world rushes onwards with the wireless revolution, Switzerland (the country that invented the World Wide Web) and the largest telecom provider, SWISSCOM – which is owned (52%) by the Swiss government – have decided to light up the public school's wired networks using fiber optics for free!
>
> But there is one catch, the schools must use LAN – local area network – with at least four connected PCs and the speed of the connection will be assigned in accordance with the number of computers linked to the school's LAN. Specifically, the Swisscom application documentation states that the schools pay for the internal wiring and connect their devices (PC, printer) via an Ethernet LAN/10BaseT/RJ45 and then connect it to a Swisscom AG's CISCO router on site. Swisscom then brings the fiber optic connection to the school.
>
> Switzerland has always had free internet access and schools could use WiFi if they wanted to. But, to get the efficiency from fiber optics, you need to use a wired LAN internet connection to get the benefit of the high bandwidth that fiber offers when hundreds of computers are streaming video at the same time. With the Internet For Schools program, the more computers that you have on your wired LAN the higher the bandwidth they provide. It's an incentive to go wired.
>
> In November 2009, Lakehead University, on the Thunder Bay campus and Orillio campus, have decided for fiber optic network, as opposed to a wireless network. Other universities have decided to remove all of their WiFi hot spots and install Ethernet connections. Hotels, that once promoted WiFi connections throughout the building, now offer Ethernet connections instead. Wired service can handle a larger volume of data transmission more rapidly, and is a more secure and reliable way of transmitting data – others can access information if wireless is used.[31]

Looking at solutions

The following is excerpted from Goldsworthy's March 2010 article, *Why Vodafone Should Not Increase the Power of Base Stations,* in response to a proposal by Vodafone that it should be allowed to increase the power of its base stations by a factor of four:

> There are now increasing reports of cancer clusters around mobile phone masts that can be attributed to a failure of the immune system to dispose of incipient cancer cells. This is the most likely explanation, since other factors that disturb our circadian rhythms, such as shift-working and exposure to continuous illumination, have similar effects on health. These include significant increases in

the incidence of breast cancer, colorectal cancer and health disorders. Similar increases are to be expected in people living close to mobile phone masts. Many of them already report poor sleep at night and tiredness during the day, which suggests that their natural circadian rhythms have been disturbed.

Present evidence suggests that *the radiation is perceived as light*, which disrupts the dark phase of the cycle, during which the immune system should be most active. If so, humans who might normally tolerate the radiation during the day, will be less able to do so at night. Every effort should therefore be made to avoid night time or continuous exposure to the radiation from base stations.

Goldsworthy suggests:

Postpone any increase in power – when you are in a hole, stop digging.

Use Femtocells. This technology uses low power domestic base stations connected to the broadband network by wired or optical links. It is already the preferred option for the mobile phone operators since it is cheaper, more reliable, and the consumer bears most of the cost. It reduces the need for investment in high power base stations and reduces the traffic through each. If Femtocells lead to the bulk of the traffic being routed through these very low power stations, which are partially shielded by the walls of the house, less will be routed through the major base stations, and the effects on the bees and other wildlife should be minimized.

The Femtocells should be no more powerful than is necessary to cover a single household and should automatically cease transmission when not in use (rather like an Orchid Low Radiation DECT Phone Base Station).

This is not just to save electricity but also to minimize disruption of the circadian rhythms and immune systems of the users, their neighbours and wildlife. The fact that most of the Femtocells would then be inactive at night when the immune system would otherwise be most active, is particularly important.

Restrict the bandwidth of the signal. A problem with digital signals is that their rapid rise and fall times generate a very large number of harmonics (multiples of the basic frequency). When these are used to modulate carrier waves, they generate very wide sidebands on either side of the carrier frequency, which actually carry the information. The width of each sideband corresponds to the frequency of the highest harmonic of the signal to be transmitted and is likely to overlap with the frequencies to which cryptochrome is sensitive. This 'out-of-band' radiation does not normally interfere with other radio transmissions because it is relatively weak at any given frequency.

However, cryptochrome is sensitive over a very wide range of frequencies and the signal is integrated over this range, so that interference may be severe. A simple solution that should be investigated is to suppress the part of the lower sideband, which overlaps with the cryptochrome range. (This is already done with analogue television, which uses vestigial sideband transmissions). The upper base station sideband, and what remains of the lower one, will still contain all the digital information, but should be relatively safe.

Other modifications: While interference with cryptochrome is probably not the only way in which modulated radiowaves from base stations give rise to biological effects, it is likely to be the one that has the most effect on the bees and also the immune system and consequent risk of cancer in human beings. Other non-thermal biological effects of mobile phone radiation, such as DNA damage, have a different aetiology, but *provided the immune system is fully functional*, most of the damaged cells may be eradicated before they become cancerous.

Nevertheless, it may be possible to do something about this too. DNA damage is most likely due to the release of structurally-important calcium ions from cell membranes by modulated radiowaves, first noted by Bawin *et al* in 1975. There is strong evidence that this weakens the membranes and makes them more inclined to leak (Goldsworthy in *Plant Electrophysiology: Theory and Methods* Ed. AG Volkov). However, it should be possible to modify the transmitted signal to avoid these effects on membranes too. This too may be easier than you think.[32, 33]

Testing of people before and after placement of antennas — chronic stress, neurotransmitters

Rapporteur Mr Jean Huss – Parliamentary Assembly – Council of Europe Report, Committee on the Environment, Agriculture and Local and Regional Affairs stated:

According to these epidemiological and also partly clinical studies, symptoms appearing or increasing sometime after relay antennas were commissioned, or after the beams emitted were intensified by raising the number or the power of the antennas, were sleeping disorders, headaches, blood pressure problems, dizziness, skin trouble and allergies. The scientific value of such local studies is regularly queried by the operators and very often the security and regulatory bodies too, and so a most recent study released early in 2011 in a German medical publication (Umwelt-Medizin-Gesellschaft 1/2011) is nonetheless worthwhile and revealing, although the number of participants in the study (60 persons) remains quite small.

These persons, from the locality of Rimbach in Bavaria, underwent analysis before a new relay antenna base station came into service in January 2004, then afterwards in July 2004, January 2005 and July 2005. In this study, as in similar epidemiological studies, the symptoms that increased or became aggravated after the station began operating were sleep disorders, headaches, allergies, dizziness and concentration problems.

The worth of this study, spanning a year and a half, is that the doctors and scientists could measure and determine significant changes in concentrations of certain stress-related or other hormones in urine samples. To sum up the results, there is a significant increase of adrenalin and noradrenalin over several months and a significant reduction of dopamine and phenylethylamine (PEA), changes indicating a state of chronic stress which, according to the authors of the study, caused the aforesaid heightened symptoms. The authors correlate the lowered PEA levels with impaired attention and hyperactivity of children, disorders which hugely increased in Germany over the years 1990-2004.

Here, too, the rapporteur stresses that some people may be more sensitive than others to electromagnetic radiation or waves. The research performed, for instance, by professor Dominique Belpomme, President of the Association for Research and Treatments Against Cancer (ARTAC), on more than 200 people describing themselves as 'electrosensitive' succeeded, with corroborative results of clinical and biological analyses, in proving that there was such a syndrome of intolerance to electromagnetic fields across the whole spectrum of frequencies.

According to these results, not only proximity to the sources of electromagnetic emissions was influential, but also the time of exposure and often concomitant exposure to chemicals or to (heavy) metals present in human tissues. In this context, Sweden has granted sufferers from electromagnetic hypersensitivity the status of persons with reduced capacity so that they receive suitable protection.

In connection with the proven or potential risks of electromagnetic fields, it should also be noted that after a Lloyd's report, insurance companies tended to withhold coverage for risks linked with electromagnetic fields under civil liability policies, in the same way as, for example, genetically modified organisms.

Finally, the rapporteur wonders whether it might not be expedient and innovative to try and develop new wireless communication technologies, equally powerful but more energy-efficient and, above all, less problematic in terms of the environment and health than the present microwave-based wireless communication. Such systems, optical or optoelectronic communication technologies employing visible and infrared light, are reportedly being developed in the United States and Japan and could largely replace the present technologies. Should such changes in transmission and communication systems prove realistic, it would then be a case of technological and economic innovations not to be missed or obstructed.[34]

WiFi caution

An open letter by Dr Magda Havas to libraries on the interference with medical devices and potential health effects of WiFi services:

DR MAGDA HAVAS, BSC, PHD

Environmental & Resource Studies, Trent University, Peterborough, ON, Canada, K9J 7B8 Phone: (705) 748-1011 x7882 Fax: (705) 748-1569
email:mhavas@trentu.ca
www.magdahavas.com and www.magdahavas.org

Date: January 12, 2010
To: Open letter to Librarians, Library Administrators and Visitors to Libraries.

ALERT: WiFi Hotspots in Libraries may be Harming Staff and Visitors and may Prevent Access to those with Medical Implants

While a growing number of libraries are installing WiFi hotspots for their visitors and staff, they seem not to be reading the literature on this topic related to health effects, interference with medical implants, speed of data transmission, and data security issues.

WiFi uses a microwave frequency of 2.45 GHz. This is the same frequency used in many mobile phones (cell and cordless) and these microwave frequencies have been linked to various illnesses, including cancer, reproductive problems, chronic fatigue, chronic pain, skin disorders, sleep disorders, cognitive dysfunction, tinnitus, dizziness, nausea, etc. That is one reason why the France National Library (BNF) decided to give up WiFi in 2008.

Based on reports of genetic alterations in human cells at WiFi frequencies (a study conducted at the University of Chicago, Department of Medicine, by Lee *et al.* 2005) and on an increasing number of scientific reports documenting ill effects of microwave exposure (including The BioInitiative Report), the safer route is to provide wired rather than wireless access to the internet.

While it might take years of exposure to develop cancer (as has been shown in mobile phone studies), changes in gene expression occurred within a matter of a few hours for cultured human cells under controlled laboratory conditions. Lee and colleagues noticed that 221 genes altered their expression after a 2-hour exposure and 759 genes after a 6-hour exposure at levels below thermal effects, on which guidelines are based. *If it doesn't heat your tissue, it is assumed to be safe*, according to federal guidelines in many countries. However, scientific studies are showing that this *'thermal effect assumption'* is no longer valid. Another consideration is that some people with medical implants may be adversely affected, because of radio frequency interference (RFI), and may not be able to visit libraries unless the WiFi service is turned off during their stay. This violates the Americans with Disabilities Act and similar acts in other jurisdictions.

Dr Gary Olhoeft, Professor of Geophysics at the Colorado School of Mines, brought this to my attention last November, at a presentation he gave in Golden Colorado organized by the EMR Policy Institute. Not only is he an expert when it comes to electromagnetic interference (EMI), but he is also one of 20 million Americans who has a medical implant. In his case, the implant is a deep brain stimulator, to control seizures due to Parkinson's disease. Malfunctions of deep brain stimulators may constitute a medical emergency and can be fatal. According to Dr Olhoeft, interference may prevent normal therapeutic function, reset or reprogram the device, bring damaging energy into the device or body, and cause injury including death.

Medical implants include cardiac pacemakers/defibrillators, neurostimulators, infusion pumps for diabetics, artificial hearts, metal rods to support broken bones, spinal stimulators, and hearing aids.

In addition to WiFi, there are a growing number of devices that can cause electromagnetic interference (EMI) including: cell phones, CB or ham radios, TV and radio transmitting antennas, theft detectors and security gates (airports, schools, stores, libraries), power lines, electric arc welding equipment, electricity substations and generators, cardiac defibrillators, diathermy equipment and MRI (Magnetic Resonance Imaging).

The France National Library replaced WiFi, not only because of health concerns, but because wired service can handle a larger volume of data transmission more rapidly, something that is essential for a large library with many researchers, and because it is a more secure and reliable way of transmitting data. The France National Library is not the first, and will not be the last replacing WiFi terminals with wired terminals.

The purpose of this open letter is to alert libraries considering WiFi to investigate the feasibility of using wired terminals, and for those libraries with WiFi to consider replacing them with wired service. Ignoring these issues of interference with medical devices and potential health effects will not make the problems go away.

As Aldous Huxley said, 'Facts don't cease to exist just because they are ignored.'

08

AUTISM

'Today we know that even a single exposure to low level radio frequency radiation causes damage to the DNA makeup of brain cells.'

Dr Robert C Kane – *Cellular Telephone Russian Roulette: A Historical and Scientific Perspective*, 2001

The autistic-child syndrome, first noticed in 1943 by child psychiatrist Dr Leo Kanner, has had an astonishing increase in recent years, which parallels the staggering increase in these silent and invisible EMF. Assistant professor of Neurology at Harvard Medical School, a pediatric neurologist at the Massachusetts General Hospital in Boston and director of the TRANSCEND Research Program, Dr Martha Herbert PhD states documentation of average to superior intelligence in most people with autism as well as domains of perceptual superiority, call into question the long-standing assumption that Autism Spectrum Disorders (ASD's) are intrinsically, or for the most part,-as sociated with cognitive deficits – another strike against the outdated 'deficit' or 'broken brain' model[1]

In the first few months of life the brain of the newborn infant is said to be 'plastic' because it is rapidly changing and making new connections and ana tomical arrangements. In the book *The Brain that Changes Itself,* the author, Norman Doidge MD, discusses the research of Michael Merzenich into brain plasticity. Merzenich has found that many of the symptoms of autism can be explained by the developing brain getting locked into an undifferentiated brain map prematurely.

Dr Robert O Becker cautioned as early as 1990 that the apparent onset of autism as a clinical condition in the early 1940s does coincide with the marked increase in our usage of electromagnetic energy. He believed it was vitally important to determine whether autism is the result of exposure to abnormal EMF, either during the final stages of fetal life or at the early newborn stage.

A 1982 WHO report in its summary *Effects of Ultrasound on Biological Systems* stated that '... animal studies suggest that neurological, behavioral, developmental, immunological, haematological changes and reduced fetal weight can result from exposure to ultrasound' – prenatal. Ultrasound uses non-ionizing radiation to convert high-frequency sound waves reflected from internal tissues and organs into images.

Former CSIRO scientist Dr Stan Barnett, in the 1990s, found evidence to suggest that pulsed Doppler exposure, as opposed to non-pulsed B-mode scanning exposure, could cause significant heating, up to five degrees in the fetus, particularly near the bone where the ultrasound beam is fixed onto a single point tissue. In 1993, the FDA approved an eight-fold increase in potential acoustical output of ultrasound equipment, though in 2008 warned on ultrasound videos and Doppler ultrasound heart beat monitors used for 'entertainment purposes'.

Using a simulation model, researchers at the Mayo Clinic characterized the audible effect of a typical ultrasound scanner as equal to 100 dB, equal to the sound of a subway train entering a station. The scientists urged doctors to use caution when directing the ultrasound probe and avoid the fetal ear, unless there is reason to suspect cranial or facial abnormalities. In 2005, Fatemi *et al* wrote, '... contrary to common beliefs, ultrasound may not be considered a passive tool in fetal imaging.'

Scientists at Yale, in 2006, found that exposure to pulsed ultrasound waves affects the movement of neurons in the brains of rodents. In mammals, including humans, neurons normally develop in one area of the brain and then migrate to the cerebral cortex. In this study, a small but significant number of neurons failed 'to acquire their proper position' and remained scattered inappropriately in the cortex or in white matter.[2] There is also concern that technicians may not be accurate in gauging exposure due to malfunctioning transducers.

Many are also curious as to why the so-called 'autism boom' of 1988–1989 increased rapidly at the same time in different countries, as identified by the Environmental Protection Agency (EPA).[3] The first commercial mobile phone networks started to spread across the USA in 1984. The switchover from analog (1G) to digital (2G) occurred in the early 1990s.

The younger the person exposed to radiation, the more concern there is about biological effects. Dr Cornelia O'Leary, a fellow of the Royal College of Surgeons in England, studied the possible relationship between Sudden Infant Death Syndrome (SIDS) and abnormal EMF.[4] In the late 1980s, she reported that eight such deaths occurred in one weekend (four of these within a single two-hour period), within a radius of a little over 11 kilometers of a top-secret military base where a powerful new radar unit was being tested.

According to Arthur Firstenberg, president of the Cellular Phone Task Force, and Susan Malloy, authors of the article Electrical Sensitivity, officials near Fort Dix, New Jersey in a town called Brick, were trying to understand why eight out of every 1,000 children born in Brick since 1994 are autistic. Medical professionals could not figure out the cause of the significant cases of autism. A 750,000-watt Doppler weather radar instrument had been installed in 1994 in nearby Fort Dix. The authors of the article believe that the reason for the increased cases of autism could possibly be attributed to electrical sensitivity to the emissions from the Doppler radar equipment.

As mentioned earlier, RF radiation from wireless technology that flows through the air can easily be received and carried by the electrical wiring network in our buildings, creating additional dirty electricity.

A 2007 ground-breaking scientific study published in the peer-reviewed *Journal of the Australasian College of Nutritional and Environmental Medicine* warned that wireless communication technology may be responsible for the accelerating rise in autism among the world's children.[5]

The primary author of the paper is Tamara Mariea, a certified clinical nutritionist and director of Internal Balance Inc based in Nashville, Tennessee who specialises in treating autism and who has helped over 500 autistic children since 2000. Mariea collaborated with Dr George Carlo, chairman of the non-profit Science and Public Policy Institute in the USA, the world's largest research program on mobile phone health hazards in the 1990s.

Mariea and Carlo's work revealed an autism-wireless technology connection following a series of tests on autistic children monitored during 2005 and 2006. Carlo stated:

> Although some of the increase in autism can be ascribed to more efficient di-
> agnosis by the medical community, a rise of this magnitude must have a major
> environmental cause. Our data offer a reasonable mechanistic explanation for
> a connection between autism and wireless technology ... These findings tie in
> with other studies showing adverse cell-membrane responses and disruptions
> of normal cell physiology. The EMR apparently causes the metals to be trapped
> in cells, slowing clearance and accelerating the onset of symptoms.

Autism and heavy metal

Autism is a disabling neurodevelopment disorder, whose cause is not com-pletely understood, but is understood to involve heavy-metal toxicity.

Of particular importance, in the Republic of Kazakhstan, metallurgical industries have a high morbidity rate and many people become invalids.

Many exposed workers have had reduced life expectancy with people often dying by the age of 50. Workers in the metallurgical industries associated with electrolytic metal extraction are exposed to high EMF. Dr E Zharkinov, professor of Medicine and head of Occupational Hygiene at the Kazakhstan Scientific Center of Hygiene and Epidemiology, reports that the electrical field exposures had a synergistic, negative effect with the simultaneous heavy-metal exposure to make the situation in those industries more hazardous.[6]

Carlo also states:

> The thing that we have identified here, this mechanism with these children with autism, what is happening in general … is they have the heavy metal build up because of their vaccines. They are exposed to the information-carrying radio waves, the active transport channels close down and heavy metals like mercury get caught inside the cell. The heavy metals disrupt the talking between messenger RNA (ribonucleic acid) and DNA and you have an environmentally induced genetic change that appears in the daughter cells. This is serious and this is happening. If you do the same exposure scenario in an older person, you have symptoms that look like Alzheimer's disease.[7]

Vaccinations

In his book *Make an Informed Vaccine Decision for the Health of Your Child*, Dr Mayer Eisenstein JD, MPH, states that when the first cases of autism began to appear in the 1940s, researchers were puzzled by the high incidence of autistic children being born into well-educated and upper-class families. Eisenstein also states that scientists unsuccessfully tried to link autism to genetic factors in upper class populations. Eisenstein also comments:

> … the first cases of autism in the United States occurred shortly after the pertussis vaccine became available. When the pertussis vaccine was initially introduced during the late 1930s, only rich and educated parents were in a position to request the newest medical advancements – the free vaccines were not available in the 1940s and 1950s. However, the growing number of children suffering from this new illness directly coincided with the increasing popularity of the mandated vaccination programs that followed.

However, considering removing dirty electricity with STETZERiZER filters has shown changes in children with autism, it is pertinent to question whether dirty electricity is playing a role in autism and ASD.

The slow spread of residential electrification in the USA in the first half of the 20th century from urban to rural areas resulted by 1940 in two large populations: urban populations with nearly complete electrification, and rural populations exposed to varying levels of electrification depending on the progress of electrification in their state. The well-educated and upper class families would have been in the urban population as over 90 percent were high school graduates and nearly three-fourths of the fathers and one-half of the mothers had graduated from college. Dr Darold Treffert calculated a rate of autism of less than 1 in 10,000 during the 1950s. It took until 1956 for USA farms to reach urban and rural non-farm electrification levels. By 1966, Dr Victor Looter found the rate of autism to be 4.1 per 10,000 children.

Slowly, dirty electricity weaved its way along our electrical wiring, assaulting our bodies, riding along the wiring in our walls not only in our workplaces but also behind our bodies, particularly our heads, where we are sleeping.

Eisenstein reports that during the 1980s and 1990s, cases of autism soared again. The increase in the levels of dirty electricity since the oil embargo of 1973 also parallels the staggering increase in autism.

Also, the MMR vaccine, which is the subject of continued controversy, was introduced in the 1980s, as were mobile phones. USA statistics report autism rose by: 1:500 – 1997, 1:150 – 2007, 1:91 – 2009, which again parallels the rise of wireless technologies and increasing amounts of dirty electricity. The Centers for Disease Control and Prevention, USA (CDC) reports the rate of autism in eight-year-olds rose 80 percent in the six-year period from 2002 and 2008. In April 2014, the CDC reported that for all children born in 2002 the rate of autism in the USA is 1:68.

Of interest, Dr Max Wiznitzer of University Hospitals in Cleveland USA, who is an expert witness for the government against the families who file in the National Vaccine Injury Compensation Program, stated on the CNN *Larry King Live* show, The Debate Over Autism in April 2009 that 'out of ten thousand individuals in our population, there was only one child with autism in northeast Ohio, the nation's largest Amish community.'[8] Wiznitzer, who is their neurologist, also claims that a public health nurse told him that there is a very high rate of vaccination amongst the Amish population. If correct, this would be contrary to the general understanding of Amish culture.

According to Dr Heng Wang, medical director at the DDC Clinic for Special Needs Children, the autism rate for the Amish around Middlefield, Ohio is 1 per 15,000. As stated previously, the Amish live without electricity.

With dirty electricity being exposed, what also must be addressed in the debate is Eisenstein reports that in Japan from 1970–1974, there were 37 documented infant deaths following pertussis vaccinations. Doctors boycotted the vaccine and in 1975 Japanese authorities raised the age of vaccination from two months to two years. As a result, babies stopped dying unexpectedly. In fact, the Japanese mortality rate improved from 17th place to best in the world, according to observations made by scientists writing in *Pediatrics*:

The category of sudden death is instructive in that the entity disappeared fol-lowing both whole-cell and acellular vaccines when immunisation was delayed until a child was 24 months of age.[9]

Dirty electricity and heavy metal

The prestigious US Naval Medical Research Institute in 1972 reported that RF radiation redistributes metals in the body. Why this highly respected research is such a critical discovery is that dirty electricity is RF radiation. Imagine a baby receiving an immunization and returning home and being exposed to dirty electricity, particularly when they sleep. Also consider the baby being exposed to the higher frequencies of wireless baby monitors.

Are the metals being redistributed and going to the brain? The Gastro Intestinal (GI) tract is considered our 'second brain', as 70 percent of the neurotransmitters in our brain are also in the GI tract. Are the metals going to the GI tract?

Once again, we should heed the observations of the Kazakhstan Scientific Center of Hygiene and Epidemiology and the synergistic negative effect of heavy metals and EMF. Just as chemicals and radiation, on their own and in combination, can contribute to the high cancer rates, we must, as a society take steps to not only address the question of vaccination but also dirty electricity and the higher frequencies, and the consequences of synergy between these two artificially created agents.

Environmental insults

Becker comments that doctors Kathryn Nelson and Lewis Holmes, of Boston's Brigham and Women's Hospital, surveyed 69,277 newborn infants and identified 48 with major developmental malformations. Of these, 16 had no family history of such problems, and the malformations thus appeared to be the result of spontaneous mutations. Becker comments that since the infants surveyed were born during the years 1972-1975 and 1979-1985, it appears at this time that at least 30 percent of genetic developmental defects in human infants are the result of some external cause. Ionizing radiation (X-ray, for ex-ample) is one such cause. The work of Heller and Manikowska-Czerska et al suggests that abnormal electromagnetic radiation may have the same effect.

Genuis reports adverse pregnancy outcomes including miscarriage, still-birth, preterm delivery, altered gender ratio and congenital anomalies have all been linked to maternal EMF exposure. A large prospective study published in Epidemiology reported on peak EMF exposure in 1063 pregnant women around the San Francisco area. After participants wore a magnetic field detector, the researchers found that rates of pregnancy loss grew significantly with increasing levels of maximum magnetic field exposure in routine day-to-day life.

Paternal EMF exposure has also been correlated with serious potential sequelae. The development of testicular abnormalities, atypical sperm, chromosomal aberrations and offspring congenital defects have all been linked to male EMF exposure. Fathers employed in industries with higher than average EMF exposure have also been noted to have offspring with higher rates of brain and spinal cord tumors.[10]

Becker also brought attention to Vernon, New Jersey, a little town of about 25,000 where the incidence of Down syndrome cases was nearly 1000 percent above the national average. On the basis of microwave transmitters, Vernon ranked fifth in the nation behind the much larger cities of New York, Chicago, Dallas and San Francisco.

In April 2009, researchers found that DNA changes affecting genes related to early brain development are involved in as many as 15 percent of cases of autism. Hakon Hakonarson of The Children's Hospital of Philadelphia, who led the ground-breaking research stated:

> Because other researchers have made intriguing suggestions that autism arises from abnormal connections among brain cells during early development, it's very compelling to find evidence that mutations in genes involved in brain interconnections increase a child's risk of autism.

In a study in 2012 of gene expression in ASDs, Rett syndrome and Down syndrome, the author's state:

> … our results surprisingly converge upon immune and not neurodevelopmental genes, as the consistently shared abnormality in genome-wide expression patterns. A dysregulated immune response, accompanied by enhanced oxidative stress and abnormal mitochondrial metabolism, seemingly represents the common molecular underpinning of these neurodevelopmental disorders.[11]

Chromosomal changes in the germ cells or the fetus can be produced by external causes.

The Bermuda Triangle of Autism

William J Walsh PhD, in *Nutrient Power: Heal Your Biochemistry and Heal Your Brain*, states 'autism is a gene programming (epigenetic) disorder.' He further states:

> It appears the combination of undermethylation, oxidative overload, and epigenetics represents the Bermuda Triangle of autism. I believe an unfortunate convergence of these three factors is the cause of most cases of autism. In

essence, autism appears to be a gene programming disorder that develops in undermethylated persons who experience environmental insults that produce overwhelming oxidative stress.

Recent studies indicate that severe oxidative stress is a distinctive feature of autism and may be the most important barrier to achieving proper brain function. The symptoms associated with excessive oxidative stress mirror the classic symptoms of autism spectrum disorders.

Elevated oxidative stress in the womb could modify epigenetic imprinting of gene expression, alter brain development, and weaken development of lymphoid and thymic tissues needed for immune function. Continuing oxidative stress in early childhood could alter development of brain cell mini columns needed for learning, memory and other cognitive functions, could inhibit brain maturation, could impair connectivity of adjacent brain regions, could increase vulnerability to toxic metals and could alter brain neurotransmitter levels. In addition, elevated oxidative stress is associated with neurodegenerative destruction of brain cells.

Taking precaution

The BioInitiative Report 2012 states oxidative stress is gaining more and more ground as being the initial mechanism of action of EMF. Herbert states the short time course needed for biologically effective EMF/RFR 'doses' to lead to observable impacts reflects that these exposures can affect cells without obstruction (unlike many chemical agents) and create impacts within minutes.[12]

Pregnant women, working at computers in a dirty electrical field and also with the contact current flowing through their bodies, need to take precautions. Women working as check-out operators in supermarkets are standing for hours in possibly high magnetic fields, dirty electrical fields and very close to scanning equipment. If the fetus does survive hazardous situations, it may explain why the list of new mental health disorders of the children of today is growing and increasing in numbers. It is also a concern that pregnant women are often in indoor employment where they are also under artificial lighting for such long periods of time.

In utero, the fetus is believed to receive a circadian melatonin message from the mother's pineal gland via its placental transfer. Following birth, the newborn is deprived of the significant rhythm for several months during which the infant produces melatonin. The circadian melatonin cycle gradually develops, beginning at three to four months of age, and by 12 months an infant is characteristically circadian.[13] Children who die of cot death – also known as SIDS – reportedly have a poorly developed pineal gland[14] and low levels of melatonin.[15] Typically, children who die of SIDS do so at the age their melatonin rhythms should be developing. Adverse EMF exposure has the potential to impact directly on pineal gland function by interfering with melatonin production and metabolism.[16]

The pineal gland – in the exact geometric centre of the head – is the principal structure in the brain that is directly sensitive to the Earth's magnetic field. The pineal is the only endocrine organ in the body whose primary regulatory control is an environmental variable.[17]

Cherry posited that external EMF signals are detected in the brain by the pineal gland and induce alterations in the calcium ion signals, that in turn send signals to the pineal gland that alters melatonin affecting the crucial melatonin/serotonin homeostasis. Melatonin and serotonin are the primary hormones of the pineal gland.

This is why we need to protect ourselves from EMF as much as possible, particularly pregnant women and newborns, as melatonin is crucial for the orderly timing of our bodily processes, particularly reproductive processes.

The neurotransmitter serotonin, which is critical to fetal brain development, has been the most intensively studied neurochemical in relation to autism over the past few decades. Serotonin allows embryos to set up consistent left-right asymmetry (heart on the correct side, etc).

While research continues on whether antidepressants taken by the mother while pregnant (particularly in the first trimester) alter serotonin levels in the fetus, the recent findings on EMF and effects on neurotransmitter levels are also of critical importance.

Serotonin acts like a radio tower in the brain, conveying signals among cells called neurons.[18] Repeated findings of elevated platelet serotonin levels in approximately one third of children with autism has led some to believe that dysfunctional serotonin signaling may be a causal mechanism for the disorder.[19]

A recent pilot research study has shown higher rates of babies born with autism where the mothers' sleeping locations had high levels of RF electromagnetic radiation.[20]

There is some anecdotal evidence that autistic children improve if the power quality in their environment is improved. Filtering the electrical environment can improve the power quality.[21]

Blank states the baby's actual radiation exposure from a wireless baby monitor is likely more than that from a nearby mobile phone antenna. He strongly advises against the use of wireless baby monitors in the home – especially close to newborns and young babies. What will be the cost if we continue to expose the highly sensitive brain and body tissue of newborn babies so intimately to artificially created EMF? Removing the EMF factor would allow a clearer picture of autism.

Hypothyroidism

Hypothyroidism – the thyroid gland is underactive – which is believed to occur in roughly 30 percent of the autistic, has a serotonin component. In October 2013, University of Sydney endocrinologist professor Creswell Eastman stated that a growing body of evidence suggested a link between expectant mums who do not make enough thyroid hormone and ASD.

A recent Dutch study also showed pregnant women with an under-active thyroid were four times more likely to have an autistic child and autistic children had more pronounced symptoms if their mothers were severely deficient for T4 – also called thyroxine.

The most common known cause of thyroid hormone deficiency is a lack of dietary iodine. Adequate iodine levels are believed to be protective for the thyroid, breast, prostate and ovary glands, and believed to protect against ionizing radiation – fall-out from nuclear/atomic bombs.

As iodine is recommended on being exposed to ionizing radiation, and Milham and Morgan suggest that the thyroid may be more sensitive to the effects of dirty electricity, and the effects from ionizing and non-ionizing radiation appear to be the same, protection from artificial EMF in our daily lives would be prudent.

Wireless baby monitors

In 2007, Goldsworthy wrote to Sir William Stewart, chairman of Britain's Health Protection Agency:

Dear Sir William

As I guess you know, there has been considerable press publicity about a possible link between the 6000 percent increase in autism in recent years and the proliferation of mobile telecommunications and WiFi.

With hindsight, we might have expected this, since their radiations have non-thermal effects on brain function. As I explained in my article at http://tinyurl.com/2nfujj (which I believe that you read some months ago), pulsed electromagnetic radiation removes structurally-important calcium ions from cell membranes and increases their tendency to leak. When this happens in neurones, it will generate spurious action potentials to create a 'mental fog', which reduces a person's ability to perform complex functions such as driving a car. This is almost certainly the explanation for the four-fold increase in the accident rate when driving a car while using a mobile phone (even when using a hands-free type).

However, even more serious is that the same mechanism could induce autism in babies. Just after its birth, a child's brain is essentially a blank canvas and it goes through an intense period of learning to become aware of the significance of all its new sensory inputs, e.g. to recognise its mother's face, her expressions and eventually other people and their relationship to him. If these processes are disrupted by spurious action potentials, they may be hindered, not accomplished in the allotted time, and the child may then express all the symptoms of autism.

A useful analogy might be the socialisation of dogs. If puppies do not meet and interact with other dogs within the first four months of their life, they too develop autistic behavior. They become withdrawn, afraid of other dogs and strangers, and are incapable of normal 'pack' behavior. Once this four-month window has been passed, the effect seems to be irreversible (i.e. just like autism).

Whether you believe my explanation for the production of spurious action potentials is a matter for personal preference, but the brain is nevertheless an electrical organ and we should not be too surprised if it is affected by extraneous electromagnetic fields, and that the 'blank canvas' of a newborn child's brain may be particularly susceptible.

While these effects might occur in response to the general electromagnetic environment, the use of cordless digital baby alarms may put the child especially at risk due to chronic exposure from a nearby source. Is it possible to get information on any correlation between the use of digital cordless baby alarms and autism and possibly other childhood problems such as cot death? If so, and the results prove positive, it may be necessary to take these devices off the shelves and advise people not to use them.[22]

Havas comments:

Most wireless baby monitors emit microwave radiation. The base station of the baby monitor is kept near the crib while the parent takes the receiver and either wears it in a hip pocket or on a belt or places it nearby to respond to the baby's crying.

Ideally a baby monitor base station should be voice-activated, meaning that it transmits sound only when it senses a sound from the baby. This would reduce the microwave exposure of both infant and parent. However, not all voice-activated baby monitors are alike.

Voice-activation mode is very different on different monitors. Some cut the radiation – some just cut the unwanted noise. The monitors in North America are constantly emitting microwave radiation. What parents in their right mind would knowingly expose their infant to constant microwave radiation?

The Swiss Government recommends 'Blue Angel' approved baby monitors. Blue Angel is a label, like CSA (Canadian Standards Association), that means the approved baby monitors are safer for the environment, including RF and EMF radiation – except CSA does not test for microwave radiation.

There are different types of babyfon baby monitors available. The one with the lowest emissions is BM 440 ECO Plus. At a distance of 30 cm, there is no added low frequency electric field or magnetic field and the radio frequency radiation is 0.0035 microW/cm^2, compared with the market average that ranges between 0.2 and 2.0 microW/cm^2.

... Do not use systems that transmit continuously ...

Health studies on baby monitors and infants

Havas further comments:

Is there a relationship between Crib Death, Sudden Death Infant Syndrome, autism, attention deficit disorder or other neurological disorders among children who were exposed to microwave emitting baby monitors as infants? There is one scientific paper that presents: A possible association between fetal/neonatal exposure to radiofrequency electromagnetic radiation and the increased incidence of autism spectrum disorders.

In the study, it suggests links to the introduction of wireless RF (Radio Frequency) communication technologies such as baby monitors to the rise autism in the public. It states:

For several decades prior to 1980, autism incidence remained essentially invariant; reportedly at about one diagnosed case per 2000 children... RF radiation sources have become commonplace in the personal human environment from approximately 1980 to the present. Operation of an RF radiation source, such as a two-way radio, portable telephone, or a cell phone, exposes the operator to levels of RF radiation shown to be biologically active ... Passive operation, such as from an RF emitting baby monitor, is a widespread postnatal exposure ... Some of the known effects of exposure to RF radiation include cognitive impairment, memory deficit, EEG modifications, DNA damage, chromosome aberrations, micronucleus formation, fetal malformation, increased permeability of the blood-brain barrier, altered cellular calcium efflux and altered cell proliferation.

According to the Autism Society of Canada – currently 1 in 110 children are diagnosed with autism today, compared to 1 in 2000 thirty years ago, when wireless baby monitors were commercially introduced. The estimated prevalence of savant abilities in autism is 10% and the most common forms involve mathematical calculations. For history buffs – the very first wireless baby monitor was tested in 1937, on Robert John (Bob) Widlar, who became a world famous mathematical savant who exhibited a complex destructive personality disorder.

Is there a link to cancers such as childhood leukemia or nervous system tumors? Do infants sleep poorly with these monitors, as indicated by Powerwatch (UK), and is the link between an infant's erratic heart rate and exposure to these baby monitors real? We just published a paper on erratic heart rate for adults exposed to a 2.4 digital cordless phone!

At any rate, exposing infants to microwave radiation, even at very low levels is unwise. Since technology is available to provide voice-activated baby monitors – the ones that emit microwave radiation only when activated – the baby monitors that emit microwave radiation continuously should be banned – especially DECT baby monitors.

In June 2009, I submitted an Environmental Petition to the Auditor General of Canada asking that DECT phones should be banned in Canada. In this petition, I also referred to DECT baby monitors.[23]

In honor of the late Robert C Kane

Dr Kane had been actively employed in the telecommunications industry for more than 30 years. He held a BSEE from the Midwest College of Engineering, an MSEE with an emphasis in electromagnetics from the Illinois Institute of Technology and also at the Illinois Institute of Technology, and completed the full course of study and research leading to a PhD in electrical engineering with emphasis in the fields of electromagnetics and solid-state physics.

As a research scientist and product design engineer, he had been directly involved with programs and projects for the design and development of mobile phones, radio frequency mobile radios, microwave telecommunications systems, video display systems and biological effects research.

Kane's 2001 book, *Cellular Telephone Russian Roulette: A Historical and Scientific Perspective*, is compelling reading. Kane conducted the testing on Motorola mobile phone research. He recently died from a brain tumor.

Kane's 2004 article below is included, due to its importance to better understand the effects of RF EMF and the staggering rise in autism.

A possible association between fetal/neonatal exposure to radio-frequency electromagnetic radiation and the increased incidence of Autism Spectrum Disorders

Abstract

Recently disclosed epidemiological data indicate a dramatic increase in the incidence of autism spectrum disorders. Previously, the incidence of autism has been reported as 4-5 per 10,000 children. The most recent evidence indicates an increased incidence of about 1 per 500 children. However, the etiology of autism is yet to be determined. The recently disclosed data suggest a possible correlation between autism incidence and a previously unconsidered environmental toxin. It is generally accepted in the scientific community that radiofrequency radiation is a biologically active substance. It is also readily acknowledged that human exposures to radiofrequency radiation have become pervasive during the past twenty years, whereas such exposures were un-common prior to that time. It is suggested that fetal or neo-natal exposures to radiofrequency radiation may be associated with an increased incidence of autism.

Introduction

Prior to the twentieth century, the only sources of radio frequency (RF) radiation were the hyper-low levels of RF energy originating from our sun and the even lower levels of extra-solar RF noise. It is in this environment of low-level RF radiation that life on Earth developed and exists to this day.

During the 1940s, primarily as a result of research and development performed as a part of the war effort, industry and the military establishment were suc-cessful in bringing the state of RF energy generation to maturity. From that time onward, we have witnessed a broad range of commercial RF energy product applications including, most notably, broadcast FM radio, radar, television, public-service mobile communication transceivers, residential microwave ovens, and the portable cellular telephone.

Initially, the contribution of each radiating device was imperceptible when weighed against the background of incoming solar radiation. However, over the span of decades the number of terrestrial RF radiation sources, now counted in the billions, has increased to the degree that, presently, the base radiation level is many thousands of times higher than from solar RF energy impinging on the Earth.

Notwithstanding the proliferation of RF radiation sources during the early de-cades of the 'radiofrequency age', the 1940s through the 1970s, humans were seldom exposed to RF radiation at levels that might cause concern. Since the late 1970s, a number of commercial products have become ubiquitous, which provide human exposures to levels of RF radiation that are significantly higher than either of the previous or present background levels. Research reports indicate that RF exposure levels, typically encountered from some commercial products, may induce alterations of biological processes or damage to the genome.[1-13]

Concurrently, the incidence of autism diagnoses demonstrates a pronounced, approximately linear, nearly three-fold increase occurring during the last twenty years. 'The question as to when autism begins in any child remains to be answered. Some studies provide support for a prenatal or perinatal origin for autism.'[14] For several decades prior to 1980, autism incidence remained essen-tially invariant; reportedly at about one diagnosed case per 2005 children. Byrd has reported a present autism incidence of about one per 700 children.

RF radiation sources have become commonplace in the personal human envi-ronment from approximately 1980 to the present. Operation of an RF radiation source, such as a two-way radio or a cell phone, exposes the operator to levels of RF radiation shown to be biologically active. Operation of an RF radiation source also exposes others, in the near proximity, to similarly biologically active levels of electromagnetic field intensities. [15]

Some of the known effects of exposure to RF radiation include cognitive impairment, [16] memory deficit, [17] EEG modifications, [18] DNA damage, [3-12] chromosome aberrations, [6] micronucleus formation, [7, 22] fetal malformation, [1, 2] increased permeability of the blood-brain barrier, [19, 23] altered cellular calcium efflux [20] and altered cell proliferation. [21]

RF radiation exposures from residential microwave ovens are, typically, on the order of 1 milli-watt per cm^2. RF radiation exposures from cell phones range from about 0.1 to 10.0 milli-watt per cm^2. Portable two-way radios provide similar exposure levels. The scientific literature confirms that RF radiation exposures, at levels more than 1,000 times lower than described immediately preceding, or on the order of 1.0 micro-watt per cm^2, induce significant changes in biological processes or molecular repair mechanisms. [12]

During gestation, the possibility of unobservable embryonic and fetal damage is increased as mothers-to-be utilize and are exposed to the emissions from RF radiation devices. Researchers have emphatically reported that an embryo or fetus should not be exposed to radiofrequency radiation such as that emitted by the portable cell phone or portable telephone. One particular reason to avoid RF radiation exposure during pregnancy is that an embryo or fetus may not be fully protected by amniotic fluid for extended periods of time due to the natural movement of the embryo or fetus within the womb. Secondly, the pelvic structure promotes deep RF radiation penetration and that radiation can be absorbed within the developing embryo or fetus.

Other researchers have postulated that there may exist a previously unidentified environmental toxin associated with the observed increased incidence of autism. For example, the works of Byrd (California – 1999), [14] Bertrand, [24] (New Jersey – 2001), Taylor, [25] (United Kingdom – 1999), and Chakrabarti & Fombonne, [26] (United Kingdom – 2001) clearly support the proposition that the identified increased incidence of autism has an origin at about 1980: an increased incidence that has its origin established at the very time the personal RF radiation devices came into popular use – about 1980. We propose that RF radiation, a new form of exposure of the human embryo, fetus, and infant, and an acknowledged environmental toxin under many exposure conditions, may be associated with the increased incidence of autism. This proposition is further based on the fact that these radiating products are periodically and typically utilized in the embryonic, fetal and neonatal environment. RF radiation is the only known toxin, exposure to which is wholly correlated with the repeatedly documented increased incidence of autism: now reported by at least some researchers as greater than 1 per 100 newborn. [24]

– **Robert C Kane PhD**, 2004

THE RIGHT TOOL FOR THE JOB

Energy Medicine and Autism – Dietrich Klinghardt MD, PhD (www.klinghardt.org)

Portion of Electromagnetic Spectrum	Brief Description	Device for measurement	safest known range for health	measured range in my house	suggestions if you are out of safe range
DC magnetic	geopathic stress, one directional magnetic fields	compass	run it across the bed-the north pole should not change		get rid of metal bed frame, box springs or mattress coils
DC electric	static electricity	negative/ positive ions	5:4 neg:pos		ventilate the home, open windows 10 minutes daily, wear and use natural fibers
AC electric	voltage/electric fields	E field detector	less than 10 volts/meter		turn off electrical circuits within 3 feet of the bed
AC magnetic	appliances/ chargers	Gauss meter	less than 0.2 Gauss		
RF electromagnetic	dirty electricity	Stetzer meter	less than 30 Graham Stetzer units		Stetzer filters or GE filters (X10 technology)
RF electromagnetic	radio frequency communications (e.g., wireless phones, HD TV's, computers)	RF detector	should not be audible in the sleeping area (more expensive analyzers can measure mW/m2 and it should be less than 5mW/m2)		unplug computers, TV's, video games and other electronics when not in use

Be aware of your EMF environment

- Are you pregnant and sleeping in a dirty electrical field?
- Are you sleeping in an electromagnetically clean environment?
- Is your baby sleeping in an electromagnetically clean environment?
- Are you pregnant and working in a dirty electrical field?
- Are you pregnant and a check-out operator at a supermarket standing in front of a register all day or working in front of a computer all day?
- If you are pregnant and live in an apartment, is your next-door neighbor's equipment, for example – fridge, air-conditioner, network server or wireless router – on the other wall to where you sleep?

Brain tumors are now the number one cause of death in children – surpassing leukemia in 2002. This could be from one type of EMF or different combinations of: ELF EMF – Transient EMF – RF EMF.

A Father's Story — Autism

In January 2009, we installed 15 STETZERiZER filters in our home. We were interested to see if they could provide any improvement for our four-year-old son who suffers from autism. Since installing the filters, we have recognized a considerable improvement in our son's behavior. He is more open to the world around him and we see a lot of progress with his cognitive abilities. A month after we installed the filters, he started to read letters and numbers on cars and he completed the alphabet for the first time in his life. Three months later, he could speak more words and he expresses his own will (which he did not do before). Nowadays, he is also very interested in puzzles.

I am convinced that the filters are not just a pill for my own headaches (I notice that the pain disappears immediately) but they also seem to have allowed my son's brain to commence a repair process.

In my opinion, although the brain of our son still has to repair and develop further, at this rate of improvement we expect to have made up significant lost ground by the end of this year.

– **J de Hass,** The Hague, The Netherlands

09

GENES VERSUS ENVIRONMENT

'... the 20th century epidemic of the so called diseases of civilization including cardiovascular disease, cancer and diabetes and suicide was caused by electrification not by lifestyle. A large proportion of these diseases may therefore be preventable.'

Professor of Medicine Samuel Milham, MD, MPH – Washington State Department of Health, USA, Historical evidence that electrification caused the 20th century epidemic of diseases of civilization, 2009

A study of 44,788 pairs of twins from Sweden, Denmark and Finland completed in 2000 concluded that environmental factors were the initiating event in the majority of cancers.[1] The emerging field of epigenetics is looking at how environmental influences can etch chemical modifications in DNA and thus introduce lifelong changes in the activity of genes.

Cancer risk is related to DNA damage: the genes are damaged. Cells with damaged DNA either die or are repaired. If repaired properly there are no further problems. DNA that is not entirely repaired or not repaired correctly leads to changes in chromosomes and mutations that can precipitate the development of cancer. Critical genetic mutations in one single cell are sufficient to progress to cancer. Inheriting a mutated gene or having a gene mutate increases cancer risk. When the rate of damage to DNA exceeds the rate at which DNA can repair the opportunity is there for cancer to develop.

Life and our health is dependent on the health and function of the different genes that control when and how our cells grow, divide and die, a delicate timing process that is constantly occurring in our bodies. Cancer develops when there is an imbalance of cell growth and cell death. The cell cycle while in the womb and in young children however is much quicker. The faster the cells duplicate, the higher the chance that something can go wrong. DNA damage and altered cell function can accelerate tumor development.

Cancer is characterized by cell division that has gone out of control. This is why it is so very important to protect the developing child from any substance that may affect this process and it is also why women are asked if they are pregnant before they are exposed to X-rays, CT scans and mammograms.

Ionizing radiation causes cancer by directly damaging DNA and disrupting normal cellular and intracellular processes. It is acknowledged that ionizing-radiation damage to genes is cumulative over a lifetime.

With regard to non-ionizing radiation EMF research has also shown disruption of normal cellular and intracellular processes. Research indicates that the effects are cumulative and that at the gene level ELF EMF and RF EMF can cause changes in how DNA works. The effects of artificial EMF on particular genes and the build-up of defective genes due to EMF exposure have already been noticed.

Earlier research reported that childhood leukemia could be triggered while in the womb. Leukemia has presented in the children of women who worked with industrial sewing machines where exposure to magnetic fields can be very high.[2] Studies (ELF EMF) conducted in the 1980s showed birth defects in the children of exposed male workers with Becker commenting that the exposure produced abnormalities in the chromosomes of the sperm.[3]

Brain tumors and nervous-system cancers have been reported in children when fathers were exposed to high levels of EMF.[4] The children and adults of today have already been affected.

Just as women are seen to be more at risk of developing breast cancer if they have certain silent carrier genes, men are also. Most cancers – particularly breast and ovarian cancer – associated with BRCA1 and BRCA2 mutations are seen in women yet men with these mutations are also at higher risk for male breast cancer, as well as prostate and pancreatic cancer and melanoma.

The very latest and ground-breaking research is reporting that people with certain genes or defective genes could be particularly sensitive to the carcinogenic effects of non-ionizing EMF/EMR.[5] The XRCC1 gene is one of many known to help repair DNA damage. A defective variant of this gene, 'rs25489' SNP,[6] has been shown to make its carriers more likely to develop breast and prostate cancer and now leukemia. Of immense interest Mexican-Americans are much more likely to carry this SNP and it has been reported that children in Mexico City have greater exposure to magnetic fields than those in other countries, often more than 6 mG units.[7]

This combination could well explain why statistics compiled by the CDC in the United States show that Mexico has one of the highest incidences of leukemia in the world.[8]

Radiowaves and lung cancer

It is not only due to its vastness that this important health issue will dwarf the cigarette-smoking and asbestos issues combined. These artificial EMF have already been shown to enhance the damage of other toxic agents. The missing pieces of the puzzle of why there is so much cancer started to appear when Örjan Hallberg and Olle Johansson looked at cancer trends during the 20th century. These fields may also be the underlying menace in the cigarette-smoking and asbestos crises.[9] The following is taken from Hallberg and Johansson's article *Cancer Trends During the 20th Century*:

> An automated computer analysis of the age-specific incidence of lung cancer among men in Sweden points at year 1955 as the starting year for a sudden environmental change in Sweden and that this disturbance mainly affects men over sixty years of age. This method of analysis has successfully been applied to study the development of melanoma of skin in Sweden, Norway, Denmark, Finland, and the United States.[10]

What happened in Sweden in 1955? In 1955 FM radio and TV1 was introduced along with the accompanying artificially created radiowaves. Hallberg and Johansson noticed, relatively shortly after the introduction of FM radio, that people who had been smoking for many years were suddenly presenting with lung cancer. The abrupt increase was not noticed in countries where FM radio had not been rolled out. For instance, Estonia had a steep increase in cancer mortality in 1991, the year that Western FM radio frequencies were allowed and introduced all over the country. In 2002 Hallberg and Johansson found statistically that country by country – and county to county within Sweden – exposure to radiowaves appeared to be as big a factor in causing lung cancer as cigarette smoking.[11]

Radiowaves and asthma

Hallberg and Johansson observed statistics in a Swedish report, which revealed that before 1960, the asthma level was essentially zero or at a very low level and that a drastic change was made to the environment conditions around 1960 or before 1960.

The melanoma link

Also in Sweden, skin melanoma statistics started to explode from 1955-1996, an increase of more than 14 times than before 1955. A similar steep rise in melanoma mortality was also reported in Queensland, Australia when comparing 1951-1959 with 1964-1967. This increase was related to the introduction of high-power TV broadcasting transmitters. Skin melanoma has also been associated with the expansion of broadcasting networks in Sweden, Norway, Denmark and the USA.

Augustsson and Stierner presented statistics on the location of moles, melanocytes and melanoma on the human body with the highest to lowest areas in descending order being: chest and back, abdomen and buttocks, lower legs, thighs, arms, head and feet. Hallberg and Johansson believe that the induced currents from RF EMF exposure are largest at these parts of the body so the mole density should be expected to follow the same pattern.

Of interest, the increase in melanoma that has occurred since the 1950s cannot be adequately explained by environmental exposure to ultraviolet radiation. Radiowaves are bounced off the ionosphere's layers in order to get around the curvature of the Earth. Are radiowaves broadcast from Earth eroding the ozone layer from below?

Extensive research in Sweden recently confirmed that adverse electromagnetic radiation is a determinant in the development of malignant melanoma, an increasingly prevalent cancer that was uncommon until about 50 years ago. Hallberg and Johansson reported a strong association between non-ionizing radiation – FM radio, 100 MHz – and the existence of malignant melanoma of the skin.[12]

In their work Hallberg and Johansson showed how weak the connection is between lung cancer and cigarette consumption in Swedish counties. A number of counties postulated that if lung cancer mortality is normalized to melanoma of skin mortality in the same counties, a very strong correlation suddenly appears. Lung cancer mortality has a multiple correlation to both cigarette consumption and skin melanoma mortality.

They report that this indicates a common factor behind the rapidly increasing mortality rates of skin and lung cancer. A closer look at lung cancer mortality shows a development very similar to skin melanoma. Lung cancer has had an almost identical development to melanoma in Sweden, with a scale factor of 10. Further, figures of melanoma and breast cancer incidences from 40 countries show an association. They concluded that breast cancer and lung cancer are linked to skin melanoma. The large numbers involved in this analysis exclude the possibility that the results are just coincidence.

Breast and prostate cancers are correlated. People who move from low-to-high-incidence countries also increase their chances. Breast, bladder, prostate, lung, colon and cutaneous melanoma cancers are all correlated with a strong relationship between melanoma and colon cancer and between lung cancer and bladder cancer.

Hallberg and Johansson concluded that there is a common environmental stress that accelerates several cancer forms, such as colon cancer, lung cancer, breast cancer, bladder cancer and malignant melanoma.

Alzheimer's disease

Alzheimer's disease (AD) is a disease of the nervous system. The BioInitiative Report concluded there is strong evidence that long-term exposure to ELF EMF is a risk factor for Alzheimer's disease. Exposure to EMF has been studied in connection with Alzheimer's disease, motor neuron disease and Parkinson's disease. These diseases all involve the death of specific neurons and may be classified as neurodegenerative diseases.

Evidence suggests that high levels of amyloid beta are a risk factor for disease, and exposure to ELF EMF can increase this substance in the brain. There is considerable evidence that melatonin can protect the brain against damage leading to Alzheimer's disease and also strong evidence that expo-sure to ELF EMF can reduce melatonin levels. Thus it is hypothesized that one of the body's main protections against developing disease – melatonin – is less available to the body when people are exposed to ELF EMF. Prolonged exposure to ELF fields could alter calcium (Ca2+) levels in neurons and induce oxidative stress.

It is also possible that prolonged exposure to ELF EMF may stimulate neurons (particularly large motor neurons) into synchronous firing leading to damage by the build-up of toxins. Evidence for a relationship between exposure and the neurodegenerative diseases, Alzheimer's and amyotrophic lateral sclerosis (ALS) is strong and relatively consistent.[13]

There is already strong evidence that long-term exposure to EMF is a risk factor for Alzheimer's disease and the latest study conducted by doctors at Bern University's Institute of Social and Preventative Medicine in Switzerland gives further evidence. The study found that the risk of developing Alzheimer's increases the longer people live next to electricity pylons: anyone who lives within the immediate vicinity of high-voltage power lines for more than 10 years has a significantly higher risk of developing dementia or Alzheimer's.[14]

Professor Denis Henshaw of the H Wills Physics Department of Bristol University, UK stated that the paper was 'like the final piece of a jigsaw. The link between childhood leukemia and power lines is already accepted by everybody.'

Professor Egger who headed the study warns that sleeping next to a radio-operated alarm clock or living beside an electrified railway line present a similar dementia risk due to proximity of the radiation source and the strength of the electrical charge.

Hearing aids use the 2.4 GHz frequency. Is this another factor contributing to dementia?

The world today

Since electricity was first generated – when the possibility of electrocution was regarded as the only hazardous side effect – to our now wireless world, exposure to EMF and the adverse health effects ranging from fatigue to serious disease and cancer have exploded within a brief timeframe:

1900 – Electricity
1920 – AM radio
1940 – Radar
1950 – FM radio, TV
1970 – Computers
1980 – Mobile phones
2000 – WiFi, WiMAX, compact fluorescent lights

By operating our computers, Play-Stations, fax machines, printers and the like we are creating additional implications for our health.

How EMR affects the body

Due to the dramatic cancer statistics from the fallout of the atomic bombs dropped on Hiroshima and Nagasaki, ionizing radiation was the first known cause of cancer. Kane comments that X-ray radiation (ionizing radiation) exposure can lead to a variety of cancers including: leukemia, bone cancer, thyroid cancer, lung cancer, brain cancer, skin cancer and more and that the list goes on to include virtually every organ and area of the body. Even though the mechanisms of action may differ between ionizing radiation and non-ionizing radiation these same cancers are also occurring from exposure to non-ionizing radiation.

All matter is composed of atoms, which have positively charged particles (protons), neutral particles (neutrons), and negatively charged particles (electrons). The protons and neutrons are clumped together in a nucleus, and the electrons move rapidly around the nucleus like planets around the sun. By default, in a stable atom, you find equal numbers of protons and electrons – meaning that the atom is neutral and has no net charge. An ionized atom has a charge because the atom has gained or lost electrons. If the atom loses electrons, that atom is a positively charged ion; if the atom gains electrons, that atom is a negatively charged ion.

Dr Martin Blank PhD, an associate professor at Columbia University in the Department of Physiology and Cellular Biophysics, and a researcher in bioelectromagnetics, in *Overpowered: What Science Tells Us About the Dangers of Cell Phones and Other WiFi-Age Devices*, explains ionizing radiation vibrates at a very high frequency with a tremendous amount of energy. When ionizing radiation comes into contact with an atom, it can knock an electron free from its orbit around the nucleus, and the atom becomes a positively charged ion. (The electron can then attach to another stable atom, resulting in a negatively charged ion). In this way, ionizing radiation causes neutral atoms to become charged ions. Ionizing radiation causes chemical reactions that in turn cause damage to biological systems (like the molecules in the body). The risks of ionizing radiation are recognized due to this power to alter the electrical charge of atoms and create ions.

Stetzer explains in regard to Transient EMF, when it reaches frequencies above 1.7 kHz the electrons in our body become excited – begin to oscillate back and forth. In other words they leave their atom in one direction, but reverse directions again. Electrons normally do not oscillate. They just stay in orbit around their atom. It is when they leave the atom that there starts to be a current flow. The rate at which they change direction is the frequency.

An assembly of cells, as in a tissue or organ, will have certain collective frequencies that regulate important processes, such as cell division. Normally these control frequencies will be very stable. If, for some reason, a cell shifts its frequency, entraining signals from neighboring cells will tend to reinstall the correct frequency. However, if a sufficient number of cells get out-of-step, the strength of the system's collective vibrations can decrease to the point where stability is lost. Loss of coherence can lead to disease or disorder.[15]

Our bodies have neutral and ionic or charged molecules. An ionic molecule reacts to changes in charge, being either attracted or repelled by charges. When those charges are changing, this sets up an oscillation within our bodies of those charged molecules. The stronger the charge internally, the greater the vibration. When we deal with resonant frequencies we have optimal absorption of the energy and the greatest possible response. This is true for all forms of RF and for ELF as well. Water (H_2O) has optimal absorption at 2.4 GHz for example, which is why microwave ovens use this frequency: it causes the water molecule to vibrate and this vibration (friction) produces heat. There are a few limiting factors but this is basically what is happening when a living organism is exposed to oscillating external EMFs.

Goldsworthy attributes most of the health effects EHS sufferers report to a single cause: at certain frequencies, weak wireless signals – far below safety standards – pull structurally important calcium ions off our body's cell membranes, weakening and causing them to leak. Robert P Liburdy PhD found in 1992, the calcium channel is the site of field interactions.[16]

Having its meticulously balanced systems destabilized, even slightly by wireless, triggered leakage wreaks biological chaos – subverting the integrity of the body's intricate defense mechanisms and leaving it vulnerable to all manner of damage. Goldsworthy theorizes how many EHS symptoms can be explained: leaking skin cells cause rashes, tingling, numbness, burning sensations; leaking heart cells trigger potentially life-threatening arrhythmias; in the inner ear, leaking cochlear cells trigger tinnitus and leaking vestibular cells cause dizziness and other symptoms of motion sickness, including nausea.

Professor James Oschman reports calcium ions slowly leak into single thalamocortical neurons, which oscillate at 1.5–28 seconds, triggering and entraining the brain waves, which spread upward throughout the brain. Eventually the thalamic oscillations cease because of the excess calcium built up in the thalamocortical neurons.

During this 'silent phase', lasting from 5 to 25 seconds, the brain waves are said to 'free run'.[17] Oschman states it is probably during this phase that the brain waves are susceptible to entrainment by external fields. Entrainment (resonance/sympathetic vibrations) describes a situation in which two rhythms that are nearly the same frequency become coupled to each other, so that both have the same rhythm. Oschman refers to the possibility that external signals, including signals projected from the hands of an energy therapist, can entrain brain waves during the thalamic silent or 'free-run' period. He also presents evidence that the 'free-run' periods, when the brain waves are not paced by the thalamus, allow the brain's field to be entrained by external electric and magnetic rhythms, either natural or man-made.[18]

Eventually the thalamic oscillations begin again, after the cells have restored their calcium levels to the point where they are once again able to oscillate. The electroencephalographic waves spread not only throughout the brain, but throughout the nervous system (via the perineural system) and into every part of the organism. In this way, the brain waves regulate the overall sensitivity and activity of the entire nervous system, as Dr Robert O Becker contended.[19]

All communication in the body eventually takes place via subtle electromagnetic signaling within and between cells, depending on precise timing and uniform communication that is being disrupted by this artificially created electromagnetic energy. These EMF are foreign invaders and the body mounts an immune response. After such chronic immune system stimulation the immune system fatigues and fails. The membranes can be locked in the inactive state. This is often referred to as 'oxidative stress' as nutrients are unable to enter into the cell, while toxins (free radicals) are not allowed to leave.

Goldsworthy reports the biological effects our safety standards ignore reads like a guest list to Dante's inferno: DNA damage, genetic changes, breakdown in intra-cell communication, protein damage, immunological function changes, reproductive system damage, decreased sperm counts, cell damage and death, brain-blood barrier leakage, brain nerve cell damage, free radical increases, melatonin decreases, possible linkage to auto-immune diseases like MS, embryonic cell damage, fetal defects, heritable birth defects, and literally hundreds of potential illnesses related to leakage in cell membranes throughout the body.

Stetzer, who is privy to the Russian research comments that the scientists working in this area state that RF radiation actually shuts down the immune system. Remove RF radiation and the body will have a chance to operate, repair, and heal more effectively.

Kane states that irritants such as asbestos or cigarette smoke residue produce a result after a long-term continual exposure. However exposures such as nuclear radiation and RF radiation are known to cause destruction and damage to tissue even with a single exposure. He also states that even a single exposure to low-level RF radiation causes damage to the DNA make-up of brain cells. Chromosomal and DNA changes occur and exposure to RF causes the alterations. The non-ionizing part of the electromagnetic spectrum, treated as harmless by many is even more of a threat as it has been woven into our whole way of living.

The impact of EMF on your cells and DNA

Blank compares our DNA to what electrical engineers refer to as a fractal antenna which receives or transmits electromagnetic radiation and is capable of picking up a range of frequencies across the electromagnetic spectrum. He explains this is why DNA is very sensitive to electromagnetic radiation – notably more sensitive to EMF than any other large molecules (such as proteins) in the body.

Electrons in DNA conduct electricity and the DNA is coiled within the nucleus. Our DNA contains different coils of different sizes that respond to many different frequencies on the EMF spectrum which explains why our DNA responds to such a wide range of frequencies. DNA is reactive across the entire electromagnetic spectrum.

According to Blank there are about 20 different stress proteins in nature called heat shock proteins (HSP) which are used by our cells to counteract harmful stimulus. Whenever a cell is exposed to an unfriendly environment the DNA separates in certain regions and begins to read the genetic code to produce these stress proteins. The presence of stress proteins is an indication that the cell has come into contact with something that is detrimental to its wellbeing. Blank states:

There's no question cells react to EMFs as harmful. Research has clearly shown that radiation within the non-ionizing range can cause single- and/or double-DNA-strand breaks which cells respond to by creating stress proteins. The reason why the DNA molecule can be made to break apart even though the radiation is non-ionizing is because of the electrical conductivity inside the DNA molecule, i.e. the electrons present in the DNA bases can be made to move. EMF's have been shown to cause electron transfer in the DNA. The idea that non-ionizing radiation cannot create a biological effect has been shown to be completely inaccurate.

Blank explains that they have now identified the DNA that controls the response to EMF. The section known as the EMF domain controls the response to EMF and by changing that part of the DNA they were able to effectively eliminate the EMF response. This particular stress protein is called hsp70.[20]

Beneficial discovery for heart patients

Blank states, as it is now known stress proteins can be induced by EMF without the need to elevate the temperature and without the need for physical contact, that this will result in increases in survival rates in cardiac bypass patients. He says exposing cardiac bypass patients to EMF has been shown to be a simpler and less damaging way to control production of hsp70 to protect the tissue from the accumulation of free radicals and oxidative damage to the tissue.

Technological advances

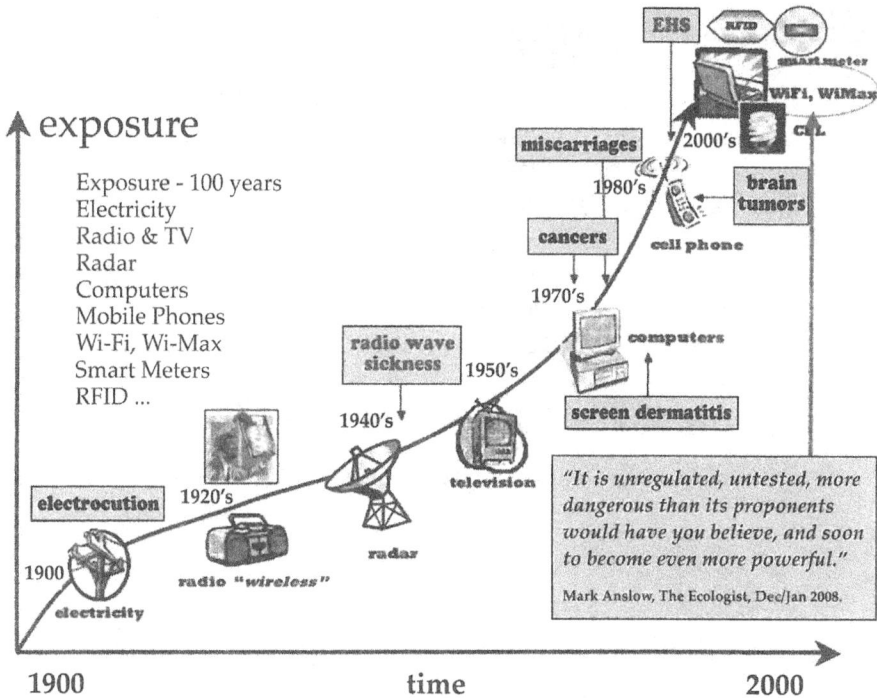

exposure

Exposure - 100 years
Electricity
Radio & TV
Radar
Computers
Mobile Phones
Wi-Fi, Wi-Max
Smart Meters
RFID ...

EHS
RFID
smart meter
WiFi, WiMax
CFL
2000's
miscarriages
1980's
brain tumors
cancers
cell phone
1970's
computers
radio wave sickness
1950's
1940's
screen dermatitis
television

electrocution
1920's
radio "wireless"
radar
1900
electricity

"It is unregulated, untested, more dangerous than its proponents would have you believe, and soon to become even more powerful."

Mark Anslow, The Ecologist, Dec/Jan 2008.

1900   time   2000

Source: Public Health SOS: The Shadow Side of the Wireless Revolution
110 Questions on Electromagnetic Pollution, from the Forum at the Commonwealth Club of California.[21]

111

Effects of Radio Frequency Fields on other organs:

- Acceleration or retardation of breathing rate
- Hemorrhaging and bleeding in internal organs
- Decreased filtration in renal tubes
- Increased activity of adrenal cortex
- Hemorrhaging in the liver
- Degeneration of hepatic cells
- Enlargement of thyroid
- Hyperthyroidism
- Increase of radioactive iodine [22]

Subjective complaints of persons working in RF field:

- Headaches
- Eyestrain
- Flow of tears
- Fatigue
- Weakness
- Disturbed sleep
- Moody
- Frequently irritated
- Unsociable
- Mental depression
- Deterioration of intellectual functions
- Notable memory impairment
- Sluggishness
- Inability to make decisions
- Loss of hair
- Muscle pain
- Pounding of heart
- Breathing difficulties
- Difficulty in sex life
- Increased perspiration of extremities
- Brittle fingernails
- Decreased lactation in nursing mothers

Symptoms of exposure to radio frequency radiation

* US Naval Medical Research Institute 1972 – declassified.[23]

Brain

- Headaches
- Dizziness
- Nausea
- Difficulty concentrating
- Depression
- Anxiety
- Memory Loss
- Muscle & joint pain
- Insomnia
- Fatigue
- Tremors
- Muscle spasms
- Tingling
- Altered reflexes

Eyes

- Pressure in/behind the eyes
- Deteriorating visions
- Cataracts

Respiratory

- Sinusitis
- Bronchitis
- Asthma
- Pneumonia

Heart

- Palpitations
- Arrhythmia
- Chest pain or pressure
- Low/high blood pressure

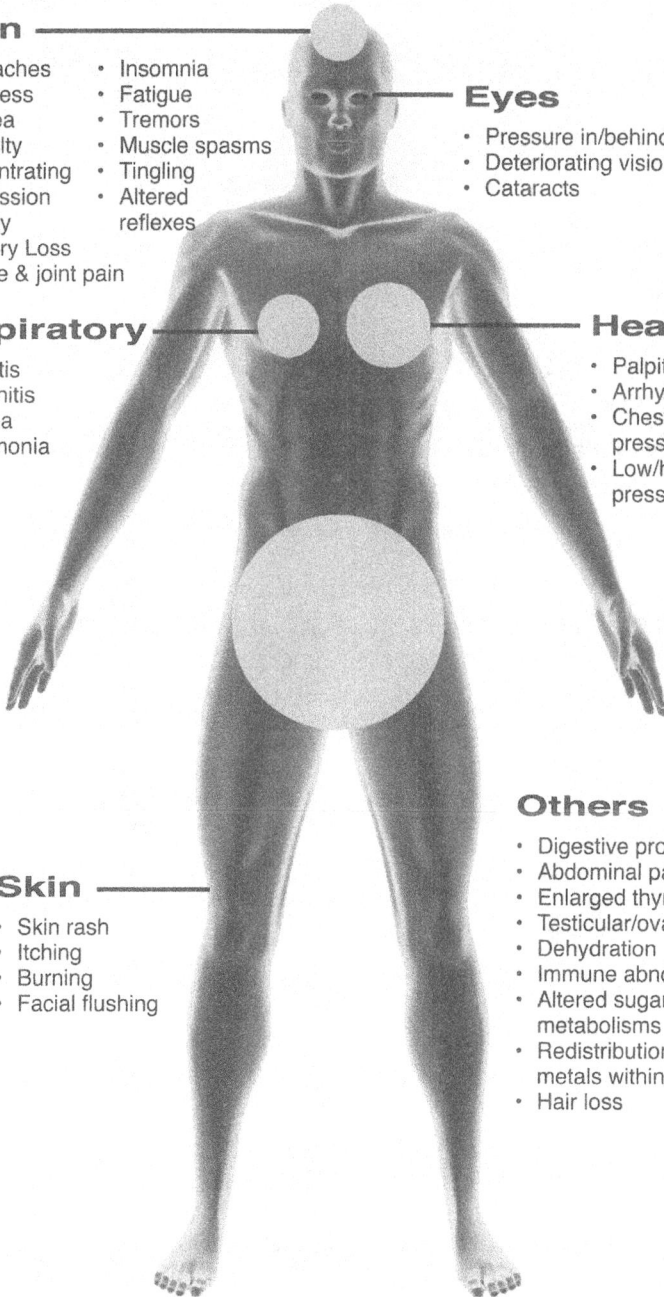

Others

- Digestive problems
- Abdominal pain
- Enlarged thyroid
- Testicular/ovarian pain
- Dehydration
- Immune abnormalities
- Altered sugar metabolisms
- Redistribution of metals within the body
- Hair loss

Skin

- Skin rash
- Itching
- Burning
- Facial flushing

(Today, also referred to as: symptoms of radio-wave sickness/EHS/exposure to dirty electricity.)

10

HOW TO MEASURE EMF

'... there is an urgent need for governments and individuals to take steps to minimize community and personal EMF exposures.'

Professor of Medicine Samuel Milham, MD, MPH
– Washington State Department of Health, USA 2008

Most employers and employees are unaware of how to address high incidences of cancer and cancers clusters in the workplace as it is difficult to understand the figures and technical language included in the reports. It is important to obtain advice from qualified private consultants who do not have a conflict of interest and are qualified in this area. Most electricians and electrical engineers are also unaware of the relevant research.

Government standards in almost all countries are inappropriately high. For example, Australia's ELF EMF standard is currently 1000 mG units for the public and 5000 mG units for occupational settings. Investigative reports quote these standards – that are the standards/guidelines for most countries – and the measurements do fall within federal guidelines.[1] It is important to understand though that these figures do not relate to the biological effects. In other words, these fields can cause disease and cancer.

In practical terms this means that you can be exposed to 499 mG units and the report will state that exposures are under the standard guidelines. You would not want to be exposed at this level for any length of time however, and it is worth noting that high fields such as these often occur. We cannot afford to remain uneducated on this topic. Fields of 2 mG units are deemed risky.

RF EMF is used when talking about emissions from broadcast, radar and wireless facilities and when describing ambient RF in the environment.

In the former Soviet Union and Eastern Europe the standards are biologically based. Most other countries base the standards on engineering computation. To date, most nations and other governing bodies that regulate power-frequency and wireless communication technologies have set safety standards based upon the heating of the skin tissue – thermal effects – and not upon the effects these waves have on the cells inside our bodies. 'If it does not heat you, it does not hurt you' is the stance that the power and telecommunications industry promotes and most radiation boards adhere to. This does not take into account the biological (cancer-causing) effects. For example, in the USA and Canada the amount of allowable RF EMF near a cell tower is one thousand microwatts per centimetre squared (1000 µW/cm²) for some mobile phone frequencies.

To help the public measure their homes, and for employers and employees to gain some knowledge on the minimum testing[2] that would be required to assess levels of workplace EMF the following suggestions are included as guidance as there can be many other problems.[3] These procedures should also be carried out in the homes of all staff, particularly in their home offices and bedrooms.

Transient EMF — Dirty Electricity
Measured in: GS units
Recommendation: Not over 40 GS units

The STETZERiZER meter should be plugged into every power outlet in the home or workplace to give a reading of the Transient EMF. This is a simple process that gives an immediate reading. The figures on the meter will keep fluctuating. This procedure should be conducted several times a day. Ideally the reading should be no higher than 30 GS units. A reading of the numeral 1 on the meter shows that the reading is over 1999 GS units. 50 GS units is approximately 2 kHz. The energy starts dissipating into the body at roughly 1.7 kHz.

In 2007 the World Health Organization (WHO) stated that acute biological effects have been established for exposure to ELF electric and magnetic fields in the frequency range up to 100 kHz that may have adverse consequences on health. Therefore, exposure limits are needed. The Republic of Kazakhstan in 2003 mandated 50 GS units for industrial purposes. It is officially recognized in Kazakhstan that there is no safe level of exposure.

Electric Field
Measured in: V/m (volts per meter)
Recommendation: less than 5 V/m

The Russian B&E meter separates the frequencies below and above 2 kHz as this is roughly the point where energy dissipates internally into the human body. The Russian standards – which does not mean 'safe' – are:

- below 2 kHz – under 25 V/m
- 2 kHz and above – under 2.5 V/m

Magnetic Field (also referred as ELF EMF)
Measured in: mG units (milligauss units)
Recommendation: 1 mG units

The Russian B&E meter can be used to measure the magnetic field which is measured in Tesla units. This meter also separates the frequencies of the magnetic field. A gaussmeter can also used although the frequencies are generally not separated. A gaussmeter measures in mG units.
   The Russian standards – which do not mean 'safe' – are:

- below 2 kHz – 250 nanoTesla = 2.5 milligauss (mG)
- 2 Khz and above – 25 nanoTesla = 0.25 milligauss

In 2001 ELF EMF was classified as an IARC 2B (possible) carcinogen.

RF EMF — Radio Frequency EMF
Measured in: microwatts per sqare centimeter – W/cm² , or volts per meter – V/m
Recommendation: 0.01 μW/cm²

The RF part of the electromagnetic spectrum is generally defined as that part of the spectrum where electromagnetic waves have frequencies in the range of around 3–300 GHz.
   The BioInitiative Report 2012 recommends for outdoor 0.003 μW/cm² as at least five new cell tower studies are reporting bioeffects in the range of 0.003 to 0.05 μW/cm². Liechtenstein mandated 0.1μW/cm² or 0.614 V/m to go into effect in 2013. The city of Salzburg limit is 0.1μW/cm².
   Measuring Equipment for RF:

- Acoustimeter: Measures – 200 MHz to 8 GHz. This meter displays green, yellow and red lights between the numerals and emits a noise.
- RF/Microwave Field Strength Analyzer HF35C: Measures – 800 MHz to 2.5 GHz. This meter displays a numerical reading and gives out noise.

There are many different RF meters available.

In 2011 RF EMF was classified as an IARC 2B (possible) carcinogen.

Contact Current
Measured in: micro Amps
Recommendation: Use a laptop in battery mode.

A Fluke 189 or 287 meter (true RMS digital multimeters) are used to conduct body current testing – contact current, induced or coupled current. Either meter measures the actual current in the body. One lead of the meter is connected directly to an EKG patch (which can be placed on the chest below the collarbone) and the other lead is connected to a single wire (which has a plug end on it, but the wire is only connected to the ground pin of the plug not the hot or neutral). Plug the wire into the electrical socket, set the meter to measure micro Amps and test.

Stetzer reports that when a person is touching the keyboard of their computer, the contact current travels along the muscle tissue up their arms until it reaches the shoulders. It follows the muscles, which spread out and go in several different directions at the chest, before reaching the legs and ultimately the floor. While this current is in the chest muscles, the breast is exposed to the hazardous current. It is known beyond doubt that breast tissue is the most sensitive tissue in the body. The fields are amplified and concentrated even more if a woman wears an underwire bra: the current/energy becomes more concentrated in this area due to the wire.

The current from the keyboard of a computer when it reaches the chest also rides down the stomach and, for pregnant women, this is very much a concern, as fetal tissue, which is very susceptible tissue, is also sensitive to artificial radiation. In Sweden, if a woman working at computers becomes pregnant, she is allowed to transfer to other duties.

It does not take much current to do some damage at the cellular level. It is believed the immune system can no longer repair the damage that the fields cause when the exposure is more than three hours. For younger people, and those not in prime health, this is a worst-case scenario.

A wise precaution is to use a laptop in battery mode only and to leave that environment while it is charging. Despite its name, placing a laptop on one's lap is not recommended.

24 micro Amps (depending on the brand) can be put into the body by touching the laptop when it is plugged in to the wall socket. 80 micro Amps will cause ventricular fibrillation in the human heart. An 11 watt compact fluorescent light – CFL – can put 27 micro Amps into the body 0.3 metres away from it.

18 micro Amps is associated with numerous well-programmed cancer studies according to the National Institute of Environmental Health and Sciences (NIEHS).

Female workers

In laboratories magnetic fields from 2–12 mG units have been found to block the action of melatonin. High levels of melatonin are associated with a lower risk of breast cancer.

These magnetic fields have also been found to partially block the action of tamoxifen, a drug routinely used for the prevention and recurrence of breast cancer. Garland in his report on the San Diego breast cancer cluster advised informing female employees about the tamoxifen research and recommended that those who were taking the drug be transferred to a lower-current area if they so desired.

More detailed information about magnetic fields, breast cancer and melatonin is available in *Silent Fields: The Growing Cancer Cluster – When Electricity Kills*.

Breast cancer cluster testimony

As more people become accurately informed they will demand to be protected in their workplaces from EMF. The following is from the testimony of associate professor Dr Magda Havas who has no conflicts of interest.

Havas submitted her testimony, *Report to the Workplace Safety and Insurance Appeals Tribunal*, for female employees of Bell Canada in Hamilton, Canada. There was a breast cancer cluster within a short period of time in this building with five breast cancers reported when 0.5 were expected. This represents a risk of 10-fold (or 900 percent increase risk) and is much higher than any of the data presented in her report except the Milham study of three breast cancers among men in a small workplace in Albuquerque, USA

Five women developed breast cancer in this workplace and three believed it to be workplace related. Havas reports that these three women were young, healthy, active with young families and no family history of breast cancer and no lifestyle habits or physiological markers that are associated with breast cancer (smoking, drinking, diet, weight, menses, parity, etc). These three women worked in front of computers and were exposed to EMF.

In her testimony Havas lists her concerns:

BFR — Brominated flame retardant

Brominated flame retardants are present in computers and are known endocrine disruptors. They are degassed from plastics and elevated concentrations are found in breast milk among women who work on computers. These brominated chemicals have been linked with higher risks of lymphoma and breast cancer (Siddiqui 2003).

CC — Contact Current

Flowing through their body from touching the keyboard. This contact current is associated with cancer at levels of 18 micro Amps (Kavet 2000) and, in conjunction with magnetic fields, generates a greater risk of cancer (Wertheimer *et al* 1995).

DE — Dirty Electricity

High voltage frequency transients – GS units

MF — Magnetic Fields

Magnetic fields – mG units

When asked the question: 'Is there any evidence that an average magnetic field of 1.86 mG could contribute to breast cancer among any or all of these three women?' Havas replied: 'yes' based on epidemiological studies of occupational exposure, on *in vivo* studies with rats showing cancer promotion, and based on *in vitro* studies showing that breast cancer 'recovery' may be compromised in a high magnetic field environment.

In her testimony Havas comments that the two women who returned to the same workplace did not survive. The woman who did not return to the same workplace survived.

In her testimony, *Breast Cancer and Occupational Exposure to Electromagnetic Fields*, Havas also states:

> In 1998 the NIEHS classified low frequency electromagnetic fields as a class 2B carcinogen based on epidemiological studies of residential exposure and childhood leukemia and occupational exposure and adult leukemia. At that time there were six studies showing an association of childhood leukemia and magnetic field exposure at values ranging from 2–4 mG. Currently there are 19 epidemiological studies showing an association between magnetic field exposure and both male and female breast cancer at values at and above 1.6 mG.

> In 1998 there were no *in vivo* studies either supporting or refuting the link between childhood leukemia and low frequency EMF exposure. In 1998 there were seven studies showing promotion of mammary tumors in laboratory animals by low frequency magnetic fields at levels between 1-500 mG. Mammary tumors in rats respond to magnetic fields and are stimulated at levels below 500 mG and are inhibited at higher exposures. In 1998 there were no *in vitro* studies either supporting or refuting the link between childhood leukemia and low frequency EMF exposure. Currently there at least six studies (independently replicated) showing that 12 mG magnetic fields promote the growth of estrogen receptor positive breast cancer (MCF-7, which is a human cell-line). These studies also show that magnetic fields reduce the oncostatic effect of both melatonin and tamoxifen.

We still do not have evidence for a plausible mechanism that explains the relationship between ELF EMF and childhood leukemia but we do have a plausible explanation for the relationship between EMF, melatonin, estrogen and breast cancer growth. In my opinion, there is little or no evidence that ELF EMF initiate breast cancer. However there is a strong body of scientific evidence showing that ELF magnetic fields promote breast cancer growth, especially estrogen-receptor positive breast cancer and that the mechanism involves inhibiting the action of oncostatic melatonin and tamoxifen. The scientific evidence for breast cancer is much stronger than it is for leukemia upon which the current classification of magnetic fields as a class 2B carcinogen was based.[4]

The 'Melatonin Hypothesis'

The Melatonin Hypothesis, theorized by Dr Richard Stevens in 1987 was based on the assumption that magnetic field exposure affects melatonin production in the same way as light-at-night and that melatonin is protective against breast cancer, possibly by affecting the level of estrogen. (Low circulating melatonin may be related directly to risk of breast cancer, or may be related through its impact on estrogen, or both, reduced melatonin levels increase the level of circulating estrogen, which would increase susceptibility to sex hormone-related cancers). The Melatonin Hypothesis is:

> Exposure to 'light at night' and/or EMF may disrupt the function of the pineal gland and its primary hormone melatonin, and that this disruption lowers melatonin production, a consequence that may lead to an increase in the long-term risk of breast cancer.

When the Melatonin Hypothesis was presented it was not known whether ELF EMF affected pineal melatonin production in experimental animals and/or humans. There was also no experimental evidence for increased breast cancer development or growth in response to ELF EMF exposure.

MRI technology

Magnetic Resonance Imaging (MRI) technology uses a strong magnetic field with pulses of RF energy. Concern is for the operators and in particular the technicians who service the machines.

RFID

RFID is radio frequency identification. Professor Konstantin Meyl, in his book *Scalar Wave Transponder*, states energy transmission occurs at around 120 kHz while information is sent back in the microwave spectrum. People in the vicinity are exposed to the sum of both scatter fields.

The Electromagnetic Spectrum

The energy from the Sun and other objects in the universe travel to the Earth in electromagnetic waves. Although the waves travel at the same speed, they may go up and down quickly (short wavelength) or slowly (long wavelength). These waves of different lengths are called the Electromagnetic Spectrum.

Visible light is part of the electromagnetic spectrum and it is the form of energy we are most familiar with because we can see it. The rest is invisible to us. With the exception of a small part of the electromagnetic spectrum from infrared through visible light, ultraviolet light and cosmic rays, the rest of the spectrum is artificial (made by humans) and foreign to human evolutionary experience.

Non-ionizing radiation includes:
artificial lighting, electrical wiring, electrical equipment/appliances, power lines, substations, mobile phones, mobile phone towers, TV and radio towers, wireless routers, RFID, MRI and smart meters.

Ionizing radiation includes:
X-rays, mammograms, CT scans, nuclear bombs.

See Appendix D for detailed Electromagnetic Spectrum illustration.

11

CLEANING UP ELECTRICITY

'The good news is that many of these EMF diseases may be preventable by simple environmental manipulation, if society chooses to pay attention. Unless public outrage intervenes, I'm afraid that our "diseases of civilization" will only get worse. Good science alone is never enough to force sensible public policy. Only citizens can do that.'

Professor of Medicine Samuel Milham, MD, MPH
– Dirty Electricity Electrification and the Diseases of Civilization, 2010

Virtually all of us are exposed to dirty electricity which flows along the streets and areas that share transformers and the power grid that ultimately supplies our power needs. Dirty electricity finds it easier to flow into the home rather than return through the transformer and onto the substation via the grid.

We are living our lives with this hazardous agent continually in our bodies. Whatever the state of the immune system an environment polluted by artificial radiation makes it weaker. It is believed that these radio frequencies use the bone marrow as their main conducting circuit within the body. The bone marrow is part of the immune system where antibodies, white blood cells and other essential 'germ fighters' are generated.[1]

Areas of risk

Manufacturers of computers are now obliged to limit the magnetic field measurements, yet the distance from dirty electricity is also a concern. Just as baby monitors can blanket a whole house with RF radiation, the frequencies from computers can blanket the entire room in call centres and workplaces that have areas of concentrated electronic equipment. Call centres are breeding grounds for higher incidences of breast cancers. Most women are unaware they are a part of a breast cancer cluster in their workplace. Prostate cancer is correlated with breast cancer, so it is equally important for men to be aware of their workplace electrical environment.

Stetzer advises that this higher-frequency field can also be concentrated in the metal chairs we sit on when working at computers, that can pose a risk for the groin area. This could be a significant factor explaining why infertility, miscarriage, birth defects, autism, altered sperm quality and quantity, cervical cancer, ovarian cancer and prostate cancers are so prevalent today.

It is critical that dirty electricity is removed from our schools, especially those with very young children. It is also critical for hospitals to install appropriate filters throughout the whole building. Shielded isolation transformers are currently installed so surgery procedure areas in hospitals are protected from these transients having a negative effect on many delicate operations, for example, heart and eye operations. It is of course essential that recovering patients – and workers – are also in an electrically clean environment.

Some anecdotal evidence suggests that people who are in cancer remission are more likely to have the cancer return if they go back to work or live in an electromagnetically hazardous environment. It also appears that malignant tissue thrives on being exposed.

Each time we purchase unfiltered electrical appliances or energy-efficient equipment and lighting we are adding to the dirty electricity plague. Ideally, electrical equipment today should be properly fitted with the appropriate built-in filter (capacitor) so the electromagnetic radiation that this equipment generates is not penetrating unsuspecting people. The cost by manufacturers to address this issue would be minimal. Appropriate filtering systems in all things electrical should be installed so their products are not only environmentally 'green' but also electrically 'clean'.

As water can become polluted when it travels through a contaminated environment so too can electricity. In our buildings the clean water comes in and the dirty water is sent out via a different pathway. Our electricity supply is contaminated, if any of the power delivered these days could indeed be considered clean. It is considered electrical pollution when it impacts equipment and electrical poisoning when it impacts living creatures.

EMF can add to and strengthen each other, multiplying instead of dividing – it depends how the supply is configured. Faulty interior wiring, poor location of electrical system elements, unacceptable current flow on water and gas lines, and electric heating coils in flooring can all heighten EMF in the home and workplace. To lessen the effects, substations need to be constructed properly and the presence of ground electrical return current on water piping addressed. Grounding errors and stray currents through water pipes can also interact with other fields. Electricity returns to Earth via the easiest route – water pipes, the return wire, Earth stake, or an unfortunate person.

Solar technology and wind turbines

Havas reports that many homes with solar panels have very high levels of dirty electricity: solar converts DC to AC with power inverters that put an enormous amount of dirty electricity on the lines and power grid.

Broadcast and mobile phone towers have their own switch-mode power supply or rectifier that converts AC to DC. Wind turbines usually change the AC to DC and the DC back to AC, a huge variable-speed frequency drive that causes enormous problems. Havas comments that another key concern is that these turbines generate both audible (noise) and inaudible (infrasound) sound waves as the human body feels and reacts to sound waves that we cannot hear. These waves, in the low end of the sound spectrum (under 20 Hz), are well documented to cause nausea, joint pain, insomnia, depression, agitation, increased blood pressure and possible heart problems. It is also a major cause of Vibroacoustic disease that can lead to vision problems, digestive problems, cardiovascular problems and circulatory difficulties.

Since infrasound can carry over very long distances, Havas states that the jury is still out on how far away from people industrial turbines should be located. Havas quotes the French Academy of Medicine guidelines that call for a minimum setback of 1.5 kilometers and Dr Nina Pierpont of New York State who has done comprehensive research into turbine-related illnesses who calls for a minimum of two kilometers. The calculation of the setback required for noise from wind turbines needs to take into consideration the change in the wind profile at night, the cyclic nature of wind turbine noise and the low frequency component of wind turbine noise.

When the dirty electricity is put on the grid it can be measured. It can also be measured on the ground for several kilometers from the source. The dirty electricity and ground current can however be eliminated with proper design.

A new electrical grid

The laws of electric engineering require that electrons flowing from a substation transformer must return to that transformer in order to complete the circuit. This is done by the use of neutral wire that exists on the distribution and transmission systems. With less than perfect grounding however this current gives rise to ground current. Because of increased load on these neutral wires more and more of the current is now completing the circuit via other routes, including the Earth and equipment.

Milham reports that much of the increase in ground current over the past 30 years is due to an aging distribution system, heavy loads on existing systems and an increasing reliance on the Earth as a conductor of that power. The transmission and distribution system in many areas cannot return such a high voltage impulse to the substation on a neutral wire.

Unfortunately the path of least resistance, which it is prone to take, is not always the straightest path. As a result it takes a path back to the substation via the ground, in streams, on metal plumbing pipes, as well as through animals and people.

When the grid was built it was designed for all current to return in the neutral wires. As the grid couldn't keep up with increasing return current loads the utilities were allowed to begin using the Earth for return currents. Over the last 20 years about 70 percent of electricity in North America returns to the substation via the Earth rather than through the neutral transmission lines. In remote sparsely populated areas, single wire Earth return systems return all current through the Earth. The recent utility practice of tying the neutral return lines to the ground also increases dirty electricity in ground currents.

Milham suggests the electric grid should be rebuilt with wiring adequate enough to return currents to the substation without using the ground. Electricity providers should remove current from the ground and put it back on the wire, *where it belongs*.

In Canada, Ontario's Legislative Assembly in 2006 passed an Act to eliminate the problem of ground current in the State, striving to eliminate ground current problems in Ontario within 10 years. It should also be possible to engineer the transients out of the electricity that is delivered to our homes and workplaces, which is essential.

In February 2009, a lawsuit was filed in the District Court in Kansas City by the United States Justice Department on behalf of the EPA. The EPA accused an energy company of failing to meet requirements of the Clean Air Act for more than a decade at a coal-fired power plant, stating that emissions from coal-fired power plants have detrimental effects on asthma sufferers, the elderly and children. These emissions have also been linked to air, water and ground pollution according to the EPA.

The government estimates that coal-fired power plants account for nearly 70 percent of all sulphur dioxide emissions and 20 percent of nitrogen oxide emissions each year. It has become obvious we need to create cleaner power in our lives from the source to the end-point. We filter our water to have cleaner water. There is no doubt that we must now filter our electricity for cleaner electricity.

As the presence of transients makes it appear that we are using more electricity than we actually are, installing filters to remove the dirty electricity should decrease power bills. The meter can also read inaccurately due to the high frequencies put on the line from the equipment at the base of mobile phone towers. Even the 25 MHz burst of energy every 1.5 seconds from strobe lights (without an RF choke) on mobile phone towers has been measured on the ground and on wires more than five kilometers away.

Exposing dirty electricity

The uncovering of the dirty electricity plague started with the problem of cows producing less milk in the 1980s. Dr Graham was an expert witness for dairy farmers who were suing milking-machine manufacturers for reduced milk production and health problems in dairy cows. He went on to patent a device for measuring and monitoring electric current flow in cows in 1995. Meanwhile, Stetzer was also an expert witness for farmers who had been dealing with similar problems in cows. He was also concerned for the families on farms who were experiencing detrimental health effects. Eventually Graham's and Stetzer's paths crossed.

Milham, in *Dirty Electricity: Electrification and the Diseases of Civilization,* acknowledges Graham and Stetzer's genius in recognizing that it was dirty electricity that was causing the problems in both cows and humans. Graham and Stetzer subsequently created the STETZERiZER meter and filters.

However it is also due to Milham's persistent attempts to expose the culprit in the La Quinta Middle School cancer cluster and by advising the teachers to file a complaint with the California Occupational Safety and Health Administration that instigated Dr Raymond Neutra's involvement and the California Department of Health Services.

It is fortunate that Milham kept persisting to have this school measured for dirty electricity. Milham still did not give up even after experiencing many closed doors and receiving a 'cease and desist' letter from the law firm Miller, Brown in Los Angeles on behalf of the new school district superintendent.

It is also fortunate for the world that Neutra knew the integrity of Graham and his work and therefore used the STETZERiZER meter to measure dirty electricity at the La Quinta Middle School. Without the efforts of these men, which also includes the efforts of Lloyd Morgan, the underlying menace as to why there is so much disease and cancer would never have been uncovered and proven.

It is essential that every Occupational Health & Safety Officer in every country is equipped with the STETZERiZER meter to protect people in their workplaces from the dirty electricity plague. Until then, we must protect ourselves at home and in our workplace and measure the levels of dirty electricity we are being exposed to and take steps to remove the dirty electricity pollution from our personal environments. Filtering our electricity will be an automatic process as more people become aware and better informed.

As filters for homes and workplaces become more widely available globally, a worldwide coalition with its roots in academia is currently being formed, acting on what the Republic of Kazakhstan immediately endorsed as valid scientific fact. Filtering our electricity is an engineering solution to an engineering problem. While filtering our electricity is not our only answer, its application is a huge step forward for civilization.

As a major contributor to the cancer story, dirty electricity is the largest threat to our health that we have ever faced as it is very much a part of our daily lives. It is in our homes, our workplaces, our schools and our hospitals. It is everywhere. This dirty electricity plague is bigger than all of us.

The scientific evidence

In his book *Cross Currents: The Perils of Electropollution, The Promise of Electromedicine*, Dr Robert O Becker details how the growth of electromagnetic pollution poses a clear danger:

> Dr Wendell Winters of the University of Texas had been contracted by the New York Department of Health to investigate the effects of 60 Hz fields on cells of the immune system. In the course of this work he had exposed human cancer cells in culture to the same fields, without specifically obtaining approval to do so.
>
> Winters reported that cancer cells increased their rate of growth by several hundred percent with only a 24-hour exposure, and that this growth rate was thereafter apparently permanent.
>
> The New York State Department of Health sent a team of investigators to Winter's laboratory. They reported that the work was not reproducible and was of questionable validity. The department also funded another investigator to 'repeat' Winter's study. This investigator reported that he was unable to duplicate Winter's results, however, he had not done the experiment in the same fashion.
>
> Work was then carried on outside the confines of the New York State study by Winters and his colleague Dr Jerry Phillips of the Cancer Research and Treatment Center in San Antonio, Texas. Winter's initial observation was confirmed and extended, leading to several recent publications in reputable, peer-reviewed scientific journals.
>
> At this time, the scientific evidence is absolutely conclusive: 60 Hz magnetic fields cause cancer cells to permanently increase their rate of growth by as much as 1600% and to develop more malignant characteristics.

These results indicate that power-frequency fields are cancer promoters – that is, they promote the growth of human cancers. The promoting effect speeds up the clinical course of any established cancer and makes it that much more difficult to treat.

Winters and Phillips worked with human cells that were already cancerous, so they could not draw any conclusions as to the possibility that these fields cause cancer. However, after surveying the entire literature on the relationship between all electromagnetic fields and cancer, doctors H D Brown and S K Chattopadhyay of the Department of Biochemistry at Rutgers University concluded that 'animal carcinogenesis studies and human epidemiological data indicate that exposure to nonionizing radiation can play a role in cancer causation.'[2]

Further investigation

Further enquiries on the study by Winters and Phillips revealed, due to the close location of the electric cord, dirty electricity would have been present. With the newer research on dirty electricity now available since this study was conducted, dirty electricity is more likely to be the cause of such an alarming conclusion: dirty electricity is not only causing cancer, it is also speeding along the progress of cancer.

Dirty electricity helps to explain the inconsistencies between the real-world studies versus the laboratory studies, where a pure 50/60 Hz sine wave is used. The graphs in Appendix C show the presence of dirty electricity and the removal of dirty electricity.

12

THE TOXIC 20TH CENTURY

'We have a history of this type of activity that delayed policy and cost millions of people their health and their lives. It happened with asbestos, with tobacco, with pesticides and is happening now with electrosmog.'

Associate professor, Dr Magda Havas, BSc, PhD
Environmental & Resource Studies, Trent University, Canada

This issue is reminiscent of the battle to clean up the cigarette smoking industry and manage the asbestos crisis and will be no stranger to inaction by authorities and governments who, as tradition has shown are slow to act on toxic agents.

Asbestos was first discovered as a cause of illness in the early 1900s but was not recognized as an occupational hazard until 1936. It was not until 1995 that a conclusive ban was placed on its use, manufacture and import.

In 1956, Dr Alice Stewart discovered that single exposures to a diagnostic X-ray shortly before birth will double the risk of an early cancer death, sparking controversy for decades.

Today it is scientific fact that exposure to ionizing radiation, even in low doses, can cause cancer. This is based on studies of Japanese bomb survivors, which showed that ionizing radiation caused the dramatic increase in breast cancer and leukemia and on studies of in-utero irradiation of the fetus.

Apart from nuclear fallout exposure to this form of radiation is by choice. The X-rays in the scanning equipment at Sydney Airport, Australia are being suggested as the cause of the current suspected breast cancer scare in airport employees.

Madan M Rehani, radiation safety specialist at the International Atomic Energy Agency (IAEA), reports it is the alarming increase in the use of high radiation dose examinations such as CT scans that is creating a need for cumulative records of patient dose, somewhat similar to the practice adopted for medical staff all these years.

Rehani states the risk of cancer from radiation doses imparted through a number of CT scans is not insignificant. On average a CT scan with 10 mSv (milliSievert) effective dose is equivalent to 500 chest X-rays, each with 0.02 mSv. Rehani also states that most other radiation effects (such as skin injury, just to name one) can be avoided rather effectively, but this is not true for the risk of cancer. He estimates a few million excess cancers in the USA over the next two to three decades from about sixty million CT scans done annually. He further reports this situation demands records of patient doses such that there is a lifetime record of how much radiation an individual has received.

A 'smart card' that contains a patient's information including radiation dose data is already in a few countries. The first meeting dedicated to the smart card project was held in Vienna in 2009. It would be prudent for more in the medical field to be recorded as well as employees in professions other than the medical field.[1]

Even though the 'mechanism of action' for how smoking causes lung cancer was not known until 1996 it was as early as 1964 when the Surgeon General's Report denounced the hazards of cigarette smoking. The efforts of whistleblower Dr Jeffrey Wiegand to expose the deceptive actions within this industry in 1996 finally prompted governments to address this issue and also the health consequences of second-hand smoke.

In 2013 the editors of *BMJ*, *Heart*, *Thorax* and *BMJ Open* decided that the journals will no longer consider for publication any study that is partly or wholly funded by the tobacco industry. The editors stated it is time to cease supporting the now discredited notion that tobacco industry research is just like any other research.[2] A similar move in regard to the power and telecommunications industries is also essential.

In 1895, the Niagara Falls Power Company opened for the first time and within a year, sent AC to Buffalo, NY, just over 25 miles (40 kms) away. Commercial AC power spread throughout the world and as a result, Nikola Tesla's high voltage coil devices which were powered by AC started to become widely known and applied. Awarded annually, the IEEE Nikola Tesla Award is one of the most distinguished honors presented by the Institute of Electrical Engineers.

In 1979, USA epidemiologist Dr Nancy Wertheimer and electrical engineer Ed Leeper in Denver, Colorado, conducted a study that resulted in worldwide attention on the link between EMF and childhood leukemia. Wertheimer and Leeper noticed in their hotly debated epidemiological research that children who were twice or three times as likely to have leukemia tended to live in homes in the Denver area close to powerlines and transformers.

Their published results found an increased incidence of childhood leukemia, lymphomas and nervous system tumors for children.[3]

Their results had an immediate effect, as in response to public opposition to the construction of new high voltage lines, the electrical industry convened an expert panel of eminent and conservative medical scientists. Included in this panel was professor David Carpenter from the New York University Department of Public Health and Dr David Savitz, one of America's most respected epidemiologists.

Carpenter's original scepticism was overturned when the Wertheimer and Leeper study, originally heavily criticized as flawed, was extended and improved. It confirmed a significantly increased risk of leukemias. Dr David Savitz reported that 20 percent of childhood cancers were attributable to exposure at 3 mG units.[4] Carpenter continued his research and is co-editor of The BioInitiative Report – 2007 and 2012.

Wertheimer and Leeper then conducted a study of adult cancer risk and their results showed that adults aged below 55 years, living long-term in residences permeated by magnetic fields of 3mG and greater, had significantly higher rates of four types of cancer due to their close proximity to high current carrying electrical powerlines. These were cancers of the nervous system, uterus, breast and lymphomas.[5]

This research prompted thousands of studies worldwide to be conducted on the magnetic field. As far back as 1997 Erren commented: 'There are more epidemiologic studies that link cancer to ELF EMF than to environmental tobacco smoke (ETS).'[6] The IARC acknowledged ELF EMF in 2001 and RF EMF in 2011 even though many scientists believe the 2B carcinogen classifications are not adequate.

In 2003, the Republic of Kazakstan not only acknowledged Transient EMF, it immediately mandated to protect its workers on conducting the research.

No other country has addressed protecting their citizens from dirty electricity as yet, even though the individuals within governments and the organizations designed to protect the people are also being exposed. Not all people choose to smoke or have been exposed to X-rays or asbestos, however we are all virtually exposed to dirty electricity day and night, every day.

Shedding light on the truth

In 2006 Genuis stated:

> ... Medical history has confirmed, however, that controversy is customary when environmental issues involve sizeable economic and health implications. Havas, a pioneer in EMR research, noted that despite considerable evidence, 'asbestos, lead, acid rain, tobacco smoke, DDT, and PCBs were all contentious issues and

were debated for decades in scientific publications and in the popular press before their health effects and the mechanisms responsible were understood'. As with previous examples, there are strong political and economic reasons for wanting no adverse sequelae to EMF exposure ...

Genuis further comments that vested interests have been effective in delaying restrictive EMF legislation by injecting confusion and doubt into scientific debate, by focusing on uncertainties and by deflecting attention from harm potential. Numerous examples have been discussed in the scientific literature where claims of environmental harm have been challenged by researchers who fail to disclose covert ties to industry.

The influence of economic interests on medical journals has also been discussed extensively in recent publications, along with examples where some editors and journal staff have suppressed publication of scientific results that are adverse to the interests of industry. In the area of adverse EMF exposure and cellular phones, for example, it has been suggested that independent study results have differed considerably from industry-funded study.[7]

Another compounding factor is that scientists cannot deliberately expose toxic compounds to humans in order to appraise what doses cause cancer. Also, Dr Carl Blackman, one of the leaders in the EMF/EMR field, reports that EMR must be treated as chemicals (plural) because we have made the mistake of treating it as a single chemical looking for single effects across the whole spectrum, when it is otherwise clear that the effects are very significant and occur at particular combinations of variables but do not occur at a nearby different combination. Blackman's work has resulted in several discoveries, including multiple effect 'windows' of intensity and frequency across the vast spectrum of non-ionizing radiation.

David Michaels, currently professor and associate chairman in the Department of Environmental and Occupational Health at the George Washington University School of Public Health and Health Services, USA, in his book, *Doubt is their Product*, explains how industry's assault on science threatens your health due to their manufacturing of uncertainty. Michaels is an epidemiologist who served as the US Department of Energy's assistant secretary for Environment, Safety and Health from 1998 to 2001 and as a regulator, saw how the USA government was manipulated by the various agencies of the government as people from industry were appointed into positions within these agencies.

Michaels explains how due to this behavior, industry were able to stop the government from regulating things that were definitely dangerous and how the government has allowed this to happen.

It is not only the public who are the victims of calculating individuals, it also our governments and doctors. *Silent Fields: The Growing Cancer Cluster – When Electricity Kills* details the challenges in delivering the landmark court case that created a world first in the EMF world. The book also details the incomplete investigation of the electrical environment regarding the breast cancer cluster at the Toowong ABC TV studios in Australia.

When professor Bruce Armstrong who led the ABC TV studio's breast cancer cluster was questioned on national TV on the frustration of some of the women who felt the proper investigations were not carried out before all the equipment was taken out he stated: 'It is very important to do the investigations properly and indeed we did have a problem with the ABC with the fairly quick decision to remove people from the site, it did mean that some of the measurements we wanted to do were not complete and I do understand how the women feel in that respect, they don't feel it's been done satisfactorily ... .'[8] The very area the women requested to be measured was not adequately measured.

Lennart Hardell PhD, Department of Oncology, University Hospital, Sweden, in his blog, January 30, 2015 encourages the public to sign a petition at:

https://secure.avaaz.org/en/petition/IARC_WHO_Move_Radio_Frequency_Radiation_from_Class_2b_to_Class_1.

Hardell's blog states:

We – the undersigned organizations, doctors, and scientists – wholeheartedly support the scientific findings of a connection between cancer and RF/EMF radiation. For the sanctity of human life, especially our children, we respectfully request that:

• WHO/IARC immediately conducts the appropriate scientific review within IARC to move RF/EMF radiation from its current class 2B to class 1, known carcinogen based on review of the complete scientific database.

• As is the policy of the WHO with smoking/cancer related issues, we respectfully request that the WHO and IARC not permit any conflicts of interests amongst the scientists, doctors, policy making/administrating officials, or anyone serving in any other capacity determining classifications of carcinogenicity and policy decisions regarding EMFs and cancer.

• Specifically we respectfully request that any scientist, doctor, policy making/administrating official, or anyone serving in any capacity in WHO and IARC not receive now or in the near future any monetary compensation from the wireless industry or any company that produces products that emit or receive RF radiation or benefit from such products or companies – in the form of research grants, consulting fees or any other form of compensation including payments to any relative of the scientist or colleague in close association.

We respectfully request that these conflicts be vehemently policed and monitored to maintain the integrity of the classifications, assure absolute transparency and ensure safety of the public.

If one is exposed to one form of artificial radiation, it would be wise to lessen exposures in other areas, that is, if we really wish to be irradiated at all. For example, the highly-respected Blank states when flying in a plane at an altitude of 20,000 feet, one is exposed to far more cosmic radiation than the body has evolved to handle, which may explain why flight crews have a higher risk of developing cancer. One of many such studies, indicated that women who have been on flight crews for more than five years have double the normal occurrence of breast cancer.[9]

We did not evolve in artificial EMF. Blank states that EMF damages and causes mutations in DNA. Mutations in DNA are believed to be the initiating steps in the development of cancers. A variety of forces, both internal and external, affects the rate at which DNA damage occurs. Blank states EMF is one of these forces, and that all EMF is bioactive.

Multiple studies have demonstrated increased rates of micronuclei in the body following exposure to radio frequency and microwave radiation.[10] A micronucleus is a fragment of DNA with no known purpose, a by-product of errors that occur during cell division.

Blank also states the presence of micronuclei indicates a type of DNA damage so strongly associated with cancer, doctors test for them as a means of diagnosing cancer.

Already it is too late for millions of women and men. Millions of dollars are raised worldwide to find a cure for cancer yet we must also take simple steps in our daily lives to lessen our bodies being irradiated. This may inconvenience us while we change societal behavior, ingrained habits and our working lives but we must not allow this to stop us from working through this together.

There should be no doubt about the validity of Dr Robert O Becker's belief that these silent EMF are a competent cause for the origin of cancers. Becker was nominated for the Nobel Prize twice due to his research in controlled EMF being used to heal.

13

ELECTROMAGNETIC HYGIENE IN 12 EASY STEPS

'Sensitivity to electromagnetic radiation is the emerging health problem of the 21st century. It is imperative health practitioners, governments, schools and parents learn more about it. The human health stakes are significant.'

William Rea, MD, Founder & Director of the Environmental Health Center, Dallas, Past President, American Academy of Environmental Medicine

Following are 12 easy steps proposed by Dr Magda Havas to create a cleaner electromagnetic environment within workplaces, at schools and in homes.

Electromagnetic Hygiene in your Workplace and School environment

1. Electric Equipment
Increase distance from electrical cords and electric equipment. Move the power bar at least 1 meter away from your feet. Use a wired extended keyboard to increase your distance from the computer screen. This will reduce the magnetic field.

2. Lighting
Try to work with the fluorescent tube lighting turned off. Remove CFL (compact fluorescent bulbs) from your work area. LED lights (ones that don't use transformers) are the lights of the future. In the meantime use incandescent light bulbs, as these do not generate poor power quality. NOTE: the original incandescent light bulbs are no longer available in Canada as the government has mandated that only energy efficient lights can be sold.

3. Internet Access

Use an Ethernet cable for Internet access (not WiFi). If you need to use wireless, ensure the wireless router is as far as possible from your body and turn it off when not in use. Ensure that you turn off the WiFi on your computer (tablet) and not just the router. Use a wired mouse and keyboard.

4. Cordless Phone

Replace your cordless telephones with a corded landline phone. The new digital cordless phones in North America (DECT phones) constantly emit microwave radiation, even when not in use. The older analog phones emit microwave radiation only when being used. The best option for reducing RF exposure is to use a wired phone.

5. Cell Phone

Text instead of talk, and use the 'speaker phone' option when talking and don't hold the phone next to your head. Do not keep phone in a pocket, in your bra, or on a belt. When signal is weak and/or phone is searching for a carrier, it is transmitting at maximum power and should not be used at this time. When not using your cell phone, keep in airplane mode (with WiFi turned off) so it does not radiate.

6. Electrical Panel & Utility Room

Ensure that workers (students) are at least 3 meters from an electric panel and are not adjacent to a utility room as these generate high magnetic fields.

Note: Low frequency magnetic fields (those that we use for electricity) can penetrate walls, windows, doors, ceilings and floors. Consequently exposure in one room may be coming from an adjacent room. For this reason it is important to spend as little time as possible near such sources even if they are on the other side of the wall. Radio frequency radiation can also penetrate walls and is blocked or reflected by metal objects generating potential hotspots. If you are in a location where there is a radio frequency (RF) source and metal objects (filing cabinet, fridge, stove, sink, etc.), your RF exposure may be higher or lower depending on the location of the source, the metal and your body.

Recommendation: Have a qualified technician measure your workplace for electrosmog. In areas where people spend hours each day, levels should be less than the following values: 1 milliGauss for power frequency magnetic fields; 5 V/m for power frequency electric fields; 40 GS units for dirty electricity; 0.01 microW/cm2 for wireless radiation; 0.5 V for ground current at 60 Hz; and 10 mV for kHz ground current.

Electromagnetic Hygiene in your Bedroom

We spend a third of each day in our bedroom and for that reason, it is important that the bedroom be electromagnetically clean. Reduce electrosmog by following the steps for your office as well as the steps below:

1. Baby Monitor

Remove wireless baby monitors. Wireless baby monitors constantly transmit microwave radiation. Infants should not be exposed to this radiation. Sound activated baby monitors are not yet available in North America but are available in Europe.

2. Clock Radio

Move clock radio (and other electric equipment) so it is at least 1 meter from your bed (clock radios emit electromagnetic fields that may affect sleep). Keep bedroom as dark as possible as light also affects sleep.

3. Computer, Cell Phone, WiFi router, tablets

Unplug computer at night if it is in your bedroom. Disconnect WiFi router and turn your cell phone off or keep it in airplane mode with WiFi turned off. This is especially important for children under the age of 18. Several national and international advisories are recommending that children under the age of 18 limit their cell phone use. Use iPods/iPads/smart tablets in airplane mode with WiFi turned off and use a wired computer for Internet access.

4. Smart Meters

Ask your utility to have your wireless smart meter wired or use analog smart meters. If this is not possible, use GS filters[1] to reduce the levels of dirty electricity generated by smart meters. Do not sleep in rooms adjacent to the smart meter. Shielding of the meter may be necessary if your smart meter emits radiation frequently (visit www.slf.co for meters and shielding material).

5. Electric Blanket and Waterbed:

Avoid use of electric blankets and waterbeds. If you need to use an electric blanket, unplug it after it has warmed the bed. This eliminates the electric and magnetic fields generated by these blankets. If you turn the electric blanket off but leave it plugged in, it will generate an electric field. So to reduce exposure unplugging the blanket is essential.

6. Turn Bedroom Power Off

Consider turning off the power (at the electrical panel) to your bedroom (and adjacent rooms) while you sleep.

Source: www.magdahavas.com – April 2004

'The greatest medical advances of the next decade will come from manipulating the body's flow of energy.'

Mehmet Oz, MD, Internationally renowned cardiac surgeon
– AARP Magazine, 2010

PART 2

LIGHT THAT HEALS

SENSING THE LIGHT

Dr A Allison, in his letter to *The Lancet*, January 10, 1880, describes a farmer who had developed cancer of the lower lip and chin. Before surgery could be performed he was struck by lightning. Alison stated:

> What seems to be the most astonishing feature in the case is the healing process which was set up in the lip and chin soon after the accident. The cancer gradually lessened, and in a few weeks every trace of the diseased structure gradually disappeared, and for ten years he enjoyed complete freedom from his former suffering and signs of the disease.

In another intriguing case in Cork, Ireland, a woman was struck by lightning and her breast cancer 'went away'. The woman had developed a hard scirrhus cancer of the breast which had resisted all treatment. (Eason 1776). She accidentally received a blow from lightning as she stood at the window during a severe thunderstorm. It set fire to the thatch roof, forced the chimney piece from the wall and raised the carpet from the floor, striking the patient on the left shoulder, across the diseased breast and down her back, burning her nightgown slightly. She remained paralysed for hours then recovered. Within two days the breast tumor had softened and diminished in size. Shortly thereafter it disappeared. The author then stated: 'Since lightning and electricity are of the same nature, should we not be encouraged to try ye electrical shock against indurated swelling glands?'[1]

Medical electricity had its golden era between the late 1700s and the early 1900s. By 1884 it was estimated that 10,000 physicians in the USA were using electricity every day for therapeutic purposes, totally without the blessing of science. By 1890, the American Electro-Therapeutic Association were conducting annual conferences on the therapeutic use of electricity and electrical devices.

Nikola Tesla

Nikola Tesla, the electrical wizard who relentlessly experimented with electromagnetic energy, is considered the father of modern electrical transmission systems and radio.

Tesla however, also created machines that flooded the human body with electrical currents and strong vibrations intended to soothe aches and promote healing. Tesla reportedly became addicted to his electrotherapeutic device, administering the treatment to himself, insisting that a session with the machine rejuvenated him on his long stretches of work without food or sleep.

Georges Lakhovsky

Georges Lakhovsky (1869–1942) was a Russian engineer, scientist, author and inventor. His controversial invention for the treatment of cancer claimed and attempted to demonstrate that living cells emit and receive electromagnetic radiations at their own high frequencies.

In 1925, Lakhovsky's philosophy was that 'the amplitude of cell oscillations must reach a certain value, in order that the organism be strong enough to repulse the destructive vibrations from certain microbes'. His remedy was not to kill the microbes in contact with the healthy cells but to reinforce the oscillations of the cell either directly by reinforcing the radio activity of the blood or in producing on the cells a direct action by means of the proper rays.

Lakhovsky's Radio-Cellulo-Oscillator (RCO) produced low frequency ELF all the way through gigahertz radiowaves with lots of extremely short harmonics. The cells with very weak vibrations, when placed in the field of multiple vibrations, find their own frequency and start again to oscillate normally through the phenomenon of resonance. Today the device is also called the Multiple Wave Oscillator (MWO). The MWO puts out a very broad spectrum of electromagnetic frequencies. Lakhovsky propounded that each cell in the body is in itself a radio receiver and works on its own special frequency. He theorized that from the bath of electrical frequencies put out by the multiwave oscillator, each cell individually could and would select the frequency which it most needed to restore its equilibrium. In simple terms, his theory was that health involved a balance or equilibrium in the electrical oscillations in living cells, and that disease arises from oscillatory disequilibrium.

Royal Raymond Rife

Royal Raymond Rife developed the Rife Universal Microscope which was capable of magnifying living cells, bacteria and even viruses up to 30,000 times their normal size so that they could be seen by the naked eye – unlike modern microscopes which look primarily at specimens that have been killed, heated and artificially stained to bring out certain cellular characteristics.

Rife's microscope used an unusual combination of quartz optics, unique in that it was able to illuminate specimens with polarized light. In the polarized light, each microorganism glowed with its own unique identifiable color.

Rife discovered each organism had its own resonant frequency – Mortal Oscillatory Rate (MOR) – and with live bacterial culture under the microscope he would turn on a frequency device known as the Rife Beam Ray that produced an EMF tuned to this (empirically derived) MOR frequency. Within moments of his turning on the field and hitting the correct frequency, all the bacteria would instantly stop moving and die.

Rife believed that the lethal frequencies for various disease organisms are coordinates of frequencies existing in the organisms themselves and that each pathogenic organism being treated is of a different chemical constituency, the consequence being they carry a different molecular vibrationary rate.

With instruments he invented that oscillated at the frequencies he had determined from the organisms, he discovered that by playing back their own pattern of oscillation, slightly modified, he could destroy them without affecting the tissues around them. Rife utilized the Rife Beam Ray on people who were infected with a specific bacterium and cured the individuals of the infectious disease. Rife found he could not only destroy common bacteria and cure chronic infections but also he could cure cancer by destroying the purported microbial causes of illnesses leaving other cells unharmed.

In 1934, Rife participated in investigational cancer research at the University of Southern California using the Rife Beam Ray, exposing 16 patients with various forms of terminal cancer to daily three-minute intervals of the MOR frequency of the BX organism. (Rife believed the cancer was caused by a virus or microorganism known as 'BX'. Dr Richard Gerber reports many cancer research laboratories have since found evidence of viral DNA in certain human cancers). Three months later, 14 of these patients were pronounced cured by a staff of five medical doctors.

Rife therapy uses the resonance effect to treat disease in a similar way to how a wine glass is destroyed when an opera singer sings at the same note (frequency). It is reported that Rife, who presented his work publicly in 1935 used pulsed EMF with a carrier wave – non-contact.

Rife observed the pH changes in what is today called the field or terrain in the microorganism's host environment as well as its association with bacterial/viral morphing.

Robert O Becker

The significant research of Dr Robert O Becker, professor of Orthopaedic Surgery at the University of New York and research surgeon at the Veteran's Administration Hospital gave evidence that electricity was a controlling factor in healing processes revealing how electrical currents within the nervous system mediate tissue repair and regeneration.

Becker examined the differences in repair between salamanders and frogs: salamanders can regrow whole new limbs from the remaining stump, whereas frogs cannot. Becker surgically amputated the arms of salamanders and then used electrodes to measure the electrical potential at the point of tissue healing. The frogs showed a positive electrical potential which gradually drifted with time to a neutral or zero potential as the stump healed over. The salamanders however, after producing an initial positive potential similar to the frogs, showed a reverse in polarity to negative potential. This negative injury potential gradually drifted back to zero over a period of days as the salamander regrew an entirely new limb. The only apparent difference between the two injury currents was that the salamander showed a swing in potential from positive to negative. Becker wondered if artificially delivering a negative potential across the frog's healing stump would affect the outcome. This he did, and to his surprise, the frog grew an entirely new limb.

Becker explained the salamander's anatomy is a duplicate of ours (or vice-versa). The salamander has the distinction of representing the basic vertebrate from which the rest of the 'higher' animals, humans included, have been derived. The salamander is capable of regrowing in full detail: a foreleg, hind leg, eye, ear, up to one-third of its brain, almost all of its digestive tract, and as much as one-half of its heart. Its growth-control systems are so effective that they also apparently prevent it from getting cancer.

Becker and his colleagues solved the riddle of why the salamander can regenerate almost anything and humans can only regenerate bone. The answer they found to what caused regenerative growth: the neuroepidermal junctions produce a negative DC current that stimulates sensitive cells in the area to dedifferentiate and form a blastema. Part of the control system that stimulates and controls regenerative growth had been identified. However, they did not know what told the blastema where it was in relation to the rest of the animal, and what it should become.

In order for a growth control system to start a healing process, it has to receive a signal indicating that an injury has occurred. Becker stated there is some mechanism within the living salamander that contains an overall plan for the salamander's body and provides the information that instructs the blastema what tissue it should construct.

Becker stated something in the process of regeneration has the ability to speak to the cancer cell and cause it to rearrange its genetic apparatus so as to deactivate the oncogenes and possibly, the signal to dedifferentiate is stronger than the oncogene signal to reproduce.

Becker also established that the meridians of the body in Chinese Medicine are skin pathways of decreased electrical resistance.

HEALER'S ENERGY

In the late 1700s, Franz Anton Mesmer theorized that subtle life-energy of a magnetic nature was exchanged between healer and patient during laying-on-of-hands. In 1969, Robert C Beck commenced research on the brain wave activity from a wide variety of healers. He found, regardless of beliefs or customs, they registered brain wave activity averaging around 7.8-8.0 Hz when in their 'healing' state. Beck also found that during the healing moments their brain waves became phase and frequency synchronized with the Schumann resonance. In the early 1980s, Dr John Zimmerman using an ultrasensitive magnetic-field detector, the Superconducting Quantum Interference Device (SQUID) magnetometer, at the University of Colorado, School of Medicine in Denver discovered that a pulsating biomagnetic field emanated from the hands of therapeutic touch (TT) practitioners. Zimmerman found the frequency of the pulsations are not steady but sweep up and down, from 0.3–30 Hz with the most activity around the Schumann resonance 7–8 Hz.

The Schumann resonance – the heartbeat of the Earth – is 7.83 Hz. The Schumann resonances are quasi-standing electromagnetic waves that exist in the Earth's electromagnetic cavity. They are the natural and vital orchestrating pulse for life on our planet sending co-ordinating signals to all organisms that connect us to the global electrostatic field. Energy for the Schumann resonance is provided by lightning. Lightning creates electromagnetic standing waves that travel around the globe, pumping energy into the Earth-ionosphere cavity, causing it to vibrate. There are on average, about 200 lightning strikes taking place every second around the planet.

In 1992, Seto and colleagues in Japan studied practitioners of various healing and martial arts techniques, including Qigong, yoga, meditation, Zen, etc. They confirmed that an extraordinarily large biomagnetic field emanates from their hands and, as in Zimmerman's study, the biomagnetic fields pulsed with a variable frequency centred around 8-10 Hz. As the biomagnetic field extends some distance from the body surface, the fields of two adjacent organisms will interact with other.

The medically established EEG brain state frequencies are: 1–4 Hz Delta, 4–7 Hz Theta, 8–14 Hz Alpha, 14–50 Hz Beta.[2] Delta activity occurs during deep sleep and in certain brain disorders. Theta activity occurs during various stages of sleep in normal adults and during emotional stresses, including disappointment and frustration. Alpha brainwaves have been associated with a normal and alert state of mind. Beta waves are normally seen over the frontal portions of the brain during intense mental activity. Beta waves of higher frequencies (up to 50 Hz) are associated with intense activation of the nervous system or tension.

Dr Richard Gerber in *Vibrational Medicine* reports studies reveal the brain-wave patterns of healer and patient both show a dominant frequency activity at 7.8 Hz and proposes the 7.8 Hz frequency is an energy window that may act in two ways to influence life.

The first is a simple transfer of magnetic energy at 7.8 cycles per second from Earth's field to the patient's energy fields. When healers enter a loving, compassionate state of increased coherence, they appear to resonantly drive the energy patterns of patients to become more coherent and ordered as well. The tendency of healing energy to create higher states of order has been suggested by research documenting the negatively entropic properties of healing energy. When healers and patients both resonate at the dominant frequency of Earth's magnetic field – the Schumann resonance – a resonance-frequency window is created. This resonance-frequency window allows energy from high potential to cascade down the magnetic waterfall of the planetary field to patients, with healers acting as conduits of that energy flow.

Gerber also suspected that the energy exchange between healers and patients is more complex than a simple transfer of magnetic energy at 7.8 cycles per second. There is, perhaps, a second function of the 7.8 Hz frequency window: the magnetic energy field may be utilized as a driving force and carrier wave for other types of energetic and frequency information being passed on to patients. In other words, the Earthfield may act as a natural waterfall of flowing energy potential. Using this analogy, the flowing water of the healer-directed Earthfield current may act as a carrier for other 'things' (such as subtle bioinformational patterns) that can be 'carried downstream'.

Gerber suggests the magnetic Earthfield may thus provide a kind of added power to the innate energy-field projection of healers, and perhaps it is the increased magnetic or magnetoelectrical currents coming from the Earthfield and cascading down through the bodies of healers that are responsible for the secondary generation of high-voltage electrical currents on the skin of healers, as was noted in Elmer Green's research. As the magnetoelectrical currents flow to patients, their energy fields undergo restructuring and repatterning that ultimately affect biochemical processes at the cellular level.

Gerber reports Dr Justa Smith found in her laboratory studies that the activity of the enzymes affected by the healers always seemed to be in a direction that was toward greater overall health and balanced metabolic activity of the organism – the direction of change in enzyme activity always seemed to mirror the natural cellular intelligence.

Dr Dolores Krieger's research demonstrated that healer's energies could increase haemoglobin levels in patients similar to the way that they increased chlorophyll content in healer-treated plants. Gerber reports this was one of the first parameters to be established which could allow quantitative biochemical measurements in humans to detect the effects of healing energy.

SIGNALS, SIGNATURES, STRESS

Today medical science uses the EEG (Electroencephalography) to measure voltage fluctuations resulting from ionic current flows within the neurons of the brain, the ECG (Electrocardiography) to measure and record the electricity activity in the heart and the EMG (Electromyography) to measure and record the electrical activity produced by skeletal muscles.

Electricity potentials and electrical currents are at all levels within the body, from the body as a whole, down to an intracellular level. Electrical potentials and electrical currents which direct and control cell behavior are generated and maintained by adenosine triphosphate (ATP), the form of energy that cells can use. Synthesis is generated by electron flow.

When tissues are diseased or damaged, the normal electrical flow and function of the body is disrupted at the cellular level – the cells experience 'their power being shut off'. Nutrients are unable to flow into the cells and toxins are unable to be released. This results in increased electrical resistance in the problem area, causing the body's electrical currents to flow around the damaged tissue. The aim of devices is to drive the current through the resistance and stimulate repair cellular regeneration.

In 2013, biologists at Tufts University School of Arts and Sciences discovered a bioelectric signal that can identify cells that are likely to develop into tumors. The researchers also found that they could lower the incidence of cancerous cells by manipulating the electrical charge across cells' membranes. 'The news here is that we've established a bioelectric basis for the early detection of cancer,' says Brook Chernet, doctoral student and the first author of a newly published research paper co-authored with Michael Levin, PhD, professor of Biology and director of the Center for Regenerative and Developmental Biology.

Levin notes, 'We've shown that electric events tell the cells what to do. The voltage changes are not merely a sign of cancer. They control and direct whether the cancer occurs or not.' Bioelectric signals underlie an important set of control mechanisms that regulate how cells grow and multiply. Chernet and Levin investigated the bioelectric properties of cells that develop into tumors in Xenopus laevis frog embryos.

In previous research, Tufts scientists showed how manipulating membrane voltage can influence or regulate cellular behavior such as cell proliferation, migration, and shape *in vivo*, and be used to induce the formation or regenerative repair of whole organs and appendages. In this study, the researchers hypothesized that cancer can occur when bioelectric signaling networks are perturbed and cells stop attending to the patterning cues that orchestrate their normal development. The Tufts biologists were also able to show that changing the bioelectric code to hyperpolarize tumor cells suppressed abnormal cell growth. 'We hypothesized that the appearance of oncogene-induced tumors can be inhibited by alteration of membrane voltage,' says Levin, 'and we were right.' Experiments to determine the cellular mechanism that allows hyperpolarization to inhibit tumor formation showed that transport of butyrate, a known tumor suppressor, was responsible.[3]

Informational signatures

Our bodies operate on the information contained in signals, whether internal or external. Two main languages are involved in communications in living systems: chemical and energetic. Energetic interactions are of two kinds: electrical and electronic. For every frequency produced by the body, there are usually harmonics and sub-harmonics (signals that are exact multiples or fractions of the 'fundamental' frequency).

Molecules and their vibrations orchestrate all living processes. Every event taking place within the body involves molecules performing tasks on other molecules and their energetic interaction is paramount. Molecules are composed of atoms, which are made up of electrons, with each electron, atom, chemical bond, molecule, cell, tissue, organ (and the body as a whole) having its own vibratory character.

Everything vibrates meaning everything is in constant motion. Life energy moves around and matter and form are modes of vibratory motion. How matter vibrates determines its form. Matter which vibrates at a very slow frequency is referred to as physical matter. That which vibrates at speeds exceeding light velocity is known as subtle matter. Subtle matter is as real as dense matter, its vibrationary (frequency) rate is simply faster.

Earthing, Electrons and Free Radicals

The body's cells face formidable threats from toxins in the foods we eat and the air we breathe, from lack of food, to infection. The body also generates free radicals as the inevitable by-products of turning food into energy and from environmental exposure. Free radicals are capable of damaging cells and genetic material and it is widely accepted that inflammation – largely caused by too many free radicals in the body – is a prime cause of a wide variety of diseases such as cancer, diabetes, heart disease, strokes, Alzheimer's and autoimmune disorders.

Our nervous system communicates using electricity, that is, movement of electrons. Molecules in our body lose an electron, become unstable, and are then classified as free radicals. With a single electron, free radicals steal electrons from any nearby substances that will yield them, for example, healthy tissues, thereby damaging them. This electron theft can radically alter the loser's structure or function. Free radicals oxidize and come in many shapes, sizes and chemical configurations.

Reducing free radicals and thus reducing disease-causing inflammation is largely a matter of getting enough electron-donors into our bodies to neutralize the free radicals. The body is constantly producing loads of molecules that quench free radicals and our bodies also extract free-radical fighters from food. These defenders, lumped together as 'antioxidants', work by generously giving electrons to free radicals without turning into electron scavenging substances themselves.

Antioxidants protect against free radicals by donating an electron to the free radical, so it no longer acts as a hungry scavenger stealing electrons from our tissues. For example, vitamin C is believed to be an electron donor. Anti-inflammatory drugs and antioxidants are electrically charged molecules that carry excess electrons to sites of inflammation where they reduce free radicals. Not all antioxidants are electron donors though. Some work through enzymatic action by preventing the formation of free radicals in the first place, by disrupting harmful biochemical processes, or by blocking free radicals from getting at healthy tissues or by physically carrying them away.

It is suggested that destructive chronic inflammation may be the result of an electron deficiency that may be remedied by contact with the Earth's infinite reservoir of negatively charged free electrons. Free electrons neutralize free radicals by donating their electrons to stablize the free radicals, making them harmless: the transfer of electrons into the body quenching or neutralizing positively charged, electron-seeking free radicals that drive chronic inflammation activity. As free electrons are natural antioxidants they do not have the disadvantages of chemical antioxidants.

In *Earthing – The Most Important Health Discovery Ever?*, Clinton Ober, Stephen T Sinatra and Martin Zucker state as exposure to sunlight produces vitamin D in the body, exposure to the ground provides an electrical 'nutrient' in the form of electrons: vitamin G – G for ground. They explain, just like the Earth, the body is mostly water and minerals and both are excellent conductors of electrons. (The natural frequencies of the Earth are waves of energy caused by the motions of subatomic particles called free electrons).

The free electrons pulsating perpetually on the surface of conductive Earth, fed by natural phenomenon – solar radiation, thousands of lightning strikes per minute, and energy generated from the planet's inner core – are easily transferred up, into, and throughout the body as long as there is direct skin contact on the ground. The authors also state that unlimited flow of electrons in the body ensures ample electrons are available in the mitochondria, and may thus contribute to the production of ATP (the fuel which gives our cells energy) in all cells.

Cardiologist Stephen Sinatra in *Earthing – The Most Important Health Discovery Ever?* states:

> ... the heart is all about ATP. The bottom line in the treatment of any form of cardiovascular disease is the restoration of your heart's supply of ATP. I've come to realize that sick hearts leak out and lose vital ATP. Cardiac conditions such as angina, heart failure, silent ischemia and diastolic dysfunction can all cause an ATP deficit.

Dr David Richards reports that he has had 25 out of 25 diabetic neuropathies resolved by placing earthing buttons over an acupuncture point called Kidney 1 (KD1) on both feet, or bands on the wrists. He has found sensation starts to return during the first session and tends to last ten days. He has not had one patient deteriorate after the initial benefit and has had three patients who have improved sensation from nerve damage after surgery.

Havas states the best way to ground is in a clean environment, walking barefoot on wet grass or along the beach. While many report benefits from earthing/grounding sheets, Havas comments a few people advised they felt 'ill' on using them. Are these the people who are the most electron-deficient? Is their environment EMF polluted? Is geopathic stress present? I have observed a few people report feeling 'ill' on using the STETZERiZER filters. When EMF is removed, Milham states the immune system is able to function more efficiently. If a detox results, adequate supplementation can support this process in people whose immune systems are compromised or damaged by EMF.

Positive and Negative Ions

Nature provides both positive and negative ions. However, our modern day way of living can remove negative ions, strip the air of negative ions or carry a high positive charge and neutralize negative ions. Environments near waterfalls, forests, or the ocean where waves break on the rocks, have an abundance of small (ingestible) negative ions of oxygen in the air. The ELANRA company states their Mk 11 ionizer replicates Nature's negative ions of oxygen, small enough to be ingested through the lungs and into the blood system within a two metre range of the needle outputs.

Geopathic stress

There is evidence to suggest that the Earth has a grid of subtle energy channels called ley lines. Earth grid lines are known as standing waves of electromagnetic energy, emanating from the ground upwards to greater heights. Some are global grids with names such as the Hartmann grid and the Curry grid.

Stressful effects upon human health, caused by abnormal fields associated with a particular geographical region, are referred to as 'geopathic stress'. Studies suggest that geopathic stress may not only contribute to illness, but may also hinder the effective treatment of disease states as well. These sites can be detected by dowsing or sensitive magnetometers with the most common cause of geopathic stress lines being underground streams.

The first notable study in recent history was conducted by Gustav Freiherr von Pohl. Research was commenced in 1922 in Central Europe following a study of unusually high cancer death rates in Vilsbiburg. A correlation between geopathic stress zones and serious illness was found when physicians compared the medical records with maps created by the dowsers. A 1989 study in Austria revealed similar results.

Gerber reports researchers have discovered the blood of normal individuals had a subtle energetic quality associated with the clockwise rotation or polarity. It has been found that individuals living in regions associated with geopathic stress tended to have a counterclockwise rotational polarity in their blood. When such individuals moved their living quarters away from these abnormal areas, their blood eventually returned to normal clockwise polarity. Clinical experience with the Vegatest system has shown that a majority of patients with cancer possess this counterclockwise blood polarity.[4]

EMF TECHNOLOGIES

Russia, Germany and Switzerland have been the leading countries using EMF for healing, using electroceuticals as opposed to pharmaceuticals. Just as the cells can be signaled to perform new and different functions by stimulation with chemicals (drugs or nutrients) they can also be signaled more robustly energetically with EMF than by chemistry.

However, in 1990 Becker cautioned about the TENS devices stating he did not believe that the potential side effects of high levels of pulsating current had been fully evaluated. Becker stopped using the devices and did not recommend their use unless all other possible techniques have been tried.[5]

TENS and Electrical Diathermy — Caution

Since the reports of an increased incidence of ALS in Italian soccer players, and US professional football players, Milham believes ALS is caused by electric currents applied to or induced in the body by exposure to TENS devices and electrical diathermy devices, because of the repeated reports of the connection of ALS with electrical shocks and electrical environments.

Electrical diathermy devices, available in the US since 1930, use shortwave radio frequency radiation and microwaves for deep tissue heating. TENS units have existed since 1974. TENS (trans-cutaneous electrical nerve stimulation) is application of electrical current through the skin for pain control.

Milham hypothesizes that sporadic ALS – 90% of cases – is caused by exogenous electrical currents induced in or applied to the body. ALS, also known as Lou Gehrig's disease, is characterized by deterioration of both upper and lower motor neurons. There is circumstantial evidence that Lou Gehrig, the famous New York Yankee baseball player who died of ALS, might have been treated with diathermy. Bob Waters, one of the three members of the 1964 San Francisco Forty-Niners professional football team who died of ALS, reported being treated for many hours with diathermy in the team's training room. At least a dozen USA and Canadian professional football players have or have died of ALS.

In August 2007, the media in Seattle, Washington carried information about Melissa Jo Ericson, a young woman who at age 28, had been recently diagnosed with ALS. She had been a basketball player at the University of Washington, followed by a professional basketball career in Europe. She was much younger than expected for this diagnosis. When Milham contacted her and inquired about her use of TENS for pain management she reported that she and her high school, college, and professional teammates had made extensive use of TENS devices provided by the schools and the professional teams.[6]

TENS — PowerTube

The advanced TENS device called PowerTube, which is used for pain therapy, is generically called a TENS device simply because it operates through transcuteneous electrical nerve stimulation. The inventor, Martin Frischknecht, states the difference to other TENS devices is that the PowerTube sends a high frequency wave signal and the output is symmetric AC current and not DC.

Frischknecht reports PowerTube homogenises the molecular cell structure of blood via three high based frequencies with a special overtone spectrum applied during therapy. This re-aligns the body's molecules and improves the internal environment. The frequencies range in the average about 200 kHz to 1.5 MHz with frequencies up to 200 MHz.

Frischknecht states the main aspect and function of the PowerTube technology is the efficient detoxification and relief from chronic and sporadic toxins within the body. Traditionally we reach for pharmaceutical medications to treat many illnesses. This introduces inorganic substances into an organic body and in the process kills important, much needed bacteria. The body is then under pressure to rid the body of these trespassers. It is also under pressure from illness and the residue of modern day preservatives and additives in our foods and chemicals in our water.

The body's energy is measurably raised at the point of re-alignment and the immune system is optimally strengthened. The result is a reinforced immune system so the body is able to fight against morbid bacteria and parasites etc, and assist with improved overall health and energy levels. Hence the body is able to heal itself. Leading research using PowerTube recently conducted by professor Dr Parlar and Dr Plichta from Germany has proven that PowerTube supports the magnetism within the cells, as magnetized iron in the blood is able to attach oxygen (O_2) to the haemoglobin which cannot be achieved using a chemical transportation process. Frischknecht states this new research confirms that PowerTube is able to bring more oxygen to cells and helps to re-alkaline the body.

Studies at the University of Munich are supporting this Swiss technology.[7]

TENS — Modulating the activity of the brain

Migraines, epilepsy, seizures, anxiety, strokes, tinnitus, ADHD, obsessive-compulsive disorder (OCD), vertigo, dysautonomia and autism

TENS devices are traditionally used for muscles. However, TENS equipment, the Chattanooga Intelect TranSport 2-Channel Electrotherapy, is currently being utilized at the Institute of Functional Neuroscience (IFN) in Australia. The IFN was established in 2008 to help improve the health and lifestyles of patients suffering from migraines, epilepsy, seizures, anxiety, strokes, tinnitus, ADHD, OCD, vertigo, dysautonomia and autism. The Institute works closely with medical and other health care practitioners to find solutions to neurologic cases that do not respond satisfactorily to established treatment protocols. It also works directly with patients for whom a medical diagnosis is inconclusive.

Functional Neurology comprises the evolving body of knowledge and clinical approach concerned with the recognition, analysis and conservative care of aberrant neurological function in the human nervous system. The clinical application of functional neurology focuses on modulating the activity of the brain that in turn changes activity throughout the nervous system. The changes that are brought about by modulating the activity of the brain are dependent on the natural processes of neural plasticity.

Neural plasticity involves activities that are fundamental to nervous system learning and functional change. IFN recognizes and uses the natural phenomenon of neural plasticity to evoke change in targeted functional areas of the nervous system. This is done in order to encourage normalization of nervous system function as far as possible. The methods utilized to evoke the neural plasticity in functional neurology tend to be conservative, non-invasive therapies.

ILLUSTRATIVE CASE STUDY

SP, a 10-year-old girl was referred to the Institute by a child psychologist with the diagnosis of ADHD. Medication had not been effective to date and the parents were now uncomfortable continuing with medication. The psychometric testing performed by the psychologist indicated that SP had diminished working memory capacity.

Working memory refers to the ability to hold and manipulate information in one's mind for brief periods of time. Most research in this area has found that working memory depends on the appropriate function of the left pre-frontal cortex. This area is essential for the coordination of recruitment of several other areas of cortex and a variety of subcortical and intrahemispheric neural networks that are also involved in this process to a greater or lesser degree depending on the nature of the information and how the information was initially perceived. The left prefrontal cortex sustains directed attention, supresses responses to irrelevant stimuli, and modulates and maintains activity in neural networks essential to completing the task at hand. Functionally, the challenge of psychometric testing may involve a lack of specificity as to which projection systems are not functioning well in the network necessary for working memory to function at the required level.

Assessment: A complete history and neurological exam was conducted as well as EEG and LORETA analysis. The results indicated that the left frontal cortex anterior cingulate system was not activating appropriately.

Treatment: Left frontal stimulus via the modalities listed below was delivered and both immediate and significant changes were observed by both the teachers and the parents over a twelve week period.

Treatment applications, imaging modalities and evidence-based references

In conjunction with standard medical diagnostics, the Institute utilizes a number of different treatment modalities, which are guided by specific imaging to stimulate brain neuroplastic changes.
Treatment Modalities:

1. Peripheral stimulation
- vibration
- manipulation (extremity and spinal)
- sound therapy
- electrotherapy (muscle stimulation and IF)
- specific exercise regimes

2. Direct current stimulation

3. Neurofeedback
- LORETA Z-score neurofeedback

4. Imaging modalities
- Quantitative EEG

Quantitative EEG and Low Resolution Electromagnetic Tomography (LORETA). LORETA is a relatively trustworthy tool for the study of brain function, and is similar to other well-established methods, such as PET and fMRI. However, unlike PET and fMRI, which provide metabolic information, LORETA images provide high time resolution electric neuronal activity information.[8]

EPRT — Electro Pressure Regeneration Therapy

EPRT Technologies USA state EPRT provides an ultra-low micro-current which recharges our cells through the use of the BodiHealth Unit, an electrical device that sends a pulsating stream of electrons in a relatively low concentration throughout the body.

In their research paper 'Ultra-Low Microcurrent in the Management of Diabetes, Hypertension and Chronic Wounds in discussing Electro Pressure Regeneration Therapy (EPRT)', Lee BY *et al* state that EPRT's action is to produce electrical pressure rather than an electrical jolt as produced by a TENS. They further state whereas a TENS device can produce a current varying from 1 μA to 100 mA, the EPRT ranges from 100 nA to 3 mA. Moreover, the TENS frequency range is from 0.5 to 40,000 Hz with a range of cycle times from 2 seconds to 0.025 milliseconds. The EPRT has a frequency of approximately 0.000732 Hz, which gives a frequency time of 22.77 minutes. Namely, a TENS with power of 10 mA and a frequency of 1 Hz is delivering approximately 6 x 10 electrons per cycle. As the cycle is one second, all these electrons were delivered in that period as a jolt. The EPRT at a setting of 100 nA is delivering 8.129 x 10 per cycle. But as this amount is being delivered over a 23 minute period (at a rate of 6 x 10 electrons per second), this behaves as a pressure instead of a jolt.[9]

In addition to its use in the treatment of diabetes and hypertension, this device is being researched for treating chronic and acute decubitus ulcers.

SCENAR

Used in Russia for over 30 years the Self Controlled Energo Neuro Adaptive Regulator – SCENAR – is the brainchild of professor Alexander Karasev working with a group of Russian scientists, engineers and physicians. This new generation of TENS is a medical technology that delivers non-invasive, non-toxic, computer modulated, and therapeutic electro-stimulation onto and through the skin.

When the electrodes of this device touch the skin, the sophisticated software automatically senses and measures electrical activity and, depending on the condition of the body, forms and sends minute electrical impulses to the body. These electrical impulses, which mimic the electrical discharges of the nervous system, stimulate the brain with a constantly changing signal that causes it to tell the nervous system to produce specific neuropeptides – the key biochemicals required by the body to regulate physiological functions and heal itself.

A Macquarie University randomized control trial in Sydney using a SCENAR personal device versus conventional TENS showed 'dramatic and sustained results' with chronic pain reduction, functional improvements and general health restoration.

Because of its effectiveness in dealing with pain, SCENAR is sometimes wrongly confused with the TENS machine which blocks pain. SCENAR which evolved from TENS stimulates the body into self-regulating away the cause of the pain.

As noted on the SCENAR Academy website in 2007, SCENAR application is indicated at any stage in treatment of the following diseases:

- nervous system (various diseases of the vertebral column with secondary disorders of the nervous activity, static and dynamic's disorders of the vertebral column, deformation of the spinal column, radiculitis, neuritis, strokes and their consequences, diseases of the vegetative nervous system, etc)
- skeletal-muscular system (myositis, arthritis, arthrosis, bruising of the soft tissue, at the fractures at different stages of the process)
- respiratory system (tracheitis, bronchitis, viral infection, pneumonia, pleurisy, bronchial asthma)
- cardio-vascular system (angina, hypertonia, hypotonia, various forms of arrhythmia), vessels of the extremities (endarteritis, varicose veins, disturbance of micro-circulation, trophic ulcers)
- digestive system (gastritis, enteritis, colitis, cholecystitis, hepatitis)
- genito-urinary system (pyeloneophritis, cystitis, disturbance of the cycle, adnexitis, infertility, toxicosis in pregnancy)
- tooth and mouth cavity diseases (peridontosis, periodontitis, arresting of inflammation and complication after the treatment of pulpitis and periodonitis, arresting pain syndrome)
- other pathological conditions and their combinations.

According to a study of 3,000 Russian medical practitioners, this device is credited with:

- 79 percent improvement in the musculoskeletal system, muscle injuries, and diseases such as arthritis, sciatica, lumbago and osteoporosis
- 82 percent improvement in many circulatory disorders, including strokes, thrombosis and heart failure

- 84 percent improvement in virtually any respiratory problems
- 93 percent improvement in both eye conditions and diseases of the digestive tract.[10]

COSMODIC

COSMODIC, also the brainchild of Karasev, differs from SCENAR in that it analyses the body's reactions on 46 components (listens to the body on 46 channels) and communicates with it allowing the device to stimulate healing on a deeper level. In simple terms, COSMODIC amplifies the body's own healing reactions.

COSMODIC is a SCENAR supplemented with biological feedback, controlled through the spectrum analysis. The spectrum of the signal makes DNA generate information which provides higher efficacy of treatment. Information from DNA, in turn, starts up mechanisms of self-regeneration – restoration of the damaged cells of the body. It has been commented it can also assist with emotional issues and deep-seated disturbances, enhancing, steering and feeding the healing potential, in a very direct manner.

PEMF

The evolution of PEMF (Pulsed Electromagnetic Field Therapy) and 'Energy Wellness' is based on physicist Michael Faraday's principle of Magnetic Induction. Studied by Jaques-Arsène d'Arsonval, understood and harnessed by Nikola Tesla, and then proven by Georges Lakhovsky, Antione Priore and Giovanni Dotto, PEMF technology is widely used today. From ultrasound and electrical stimulation, to laser or sound therapy, these scientists still have a large impact in today's world.

PEMF refers to short pulses with various wave forms. The pulse timing, interval and duration all differ depending on the manufacturer of the product. If you fracture a bone in an arm or leg and it fails to heal in 3-6 months, PEMF may be suggested. PEMF is also being used for injuries of soft tissues, such as nerve, skin, muscle, and tendon, and the pain associated with such injuries. PEMF devices tend to use Earth frequencies and their harmonics – multiples of the frequency. A common denominator is the production of pulsating magnetic fields that induce currents to flow within tissues.

James Oschman PhD, explains that the PEMF device produces a magnetic field that induces currents to flow in nearby tissues and that clinical tests have proved that PEMF therapy will 'jump start' bone repair. Medical research has revealed that magnetic fields 'can convert a stalled healing process into active repair, even in patients unhealed for as long as 40 years'.[11]

Oschman further states, not surprisingly, the scientific evidence is that PEMF therapy is effective because it conveys 'information' that triggers specific repair activities within the body. The currents induced in tissues by PEMF mimic the natural electrical activities created within bones during movements. Pulsing magnetic fields initiate a cascade of activities, from the cell membrane to the nucleus and on to the gene level, where specific changes take place. To be effective, PEMF pulses must be of low energy and extremely low frequency (ELF). Oschman reports recent research shows that comparable fields emanate from the hands of practitioners of therapeutic touch and related methods.

NASA has been testing the effect of PEMF as a countermeasure for bone loss and muscular degeneration encountered by astronauts on long space missions. Dr Thomas Goodwin and NASA have a patent for a device that uses low frequency low intensity square wave magnetic fields to enhance the rate of healing of mammalian body parts.

Dr Thomas Rau of the Paracelsus Klinik in Switzerland, a world famous clinic known for treating difficult cases uses PEMF after first performing dental procedures.[12]

Havas states there is evidence exposure to therapeutic PEMF reduces blood viscosity, improves blood circulation, benefits the immune system, promotes the healing of bone fractures, fights depression and reduces pain. PEMF devices do not treat a specific condition – they optimize the body's natural healing and self regulating mechanisms.

There has been no study of the long-term effects of PEMF devices to date, as they are a relatively new technology. Considering the information that has come to light regarding overuse of the earlier TENS devices, caution should always be used when applying current to the body, regardless of the technology.

Havas is currently studying the long-term effects of PEMF and states they are being used for:

- acid deposits
- ADHD
- aging
- allergies
- ankylosing spondylitis
- arteriosclerosis
- arthritis
- asthma
- back pain
- cardiac arrhythmia

- cardiovascular disease
- chronic fatigue
- depression
- diabetes
- fibromyalgia
- inflammatory intestinal diseases
- injuries
- lupus
- macular degeneration
- multiple sclerosis
- muscle dystrophy
- osteoarthritis
- osteoporosis
- pacemakers
- pain
- parkinson's disease
- respiratory disease
- restless leg syndrome
- rheumatic diseases
- sarcoidosis
- sports injury
- stroke
- thrombosis
- tinnitus
- trauma
- tumor
- wounds

Research into using PEMF for ASD is also being conducted. Havas reports some people who are electrically sensitive are unable to use the devices but others seem to do quite well. The reason for this is unknown.

NIIT

NIIT (Non-invasive Magnetic Induction Therapy) technology takes the good components from a lightning strike and acts as a controlled lightning strike: the induction of negative ions and exciting almost all the frequencies of the electromagnetic spectrum all at once. Likened to pressing all of the keys on a piano at once, this technology allows the body to accept which frequencies are needed. This technology is a high-powered PEMF using high-end frequencies to carry the low-end frequencies.

The frequency of energy utilized for treatment appears to be a critical element for successful therapy – the frequency of the pulsed electromagnetic fields being a key factor. This therapy uses waves of energy that pass through the cells. It is the speed of the pulse that is significant and this therapy is a very fast and instantaneous pulse. A slow pulse is a microwave. These machines use a fast pulse: too much time creates heat.

NIIT acts as a catalyst to improve various chemical reactions by enhancing the electron transfer rate. Electron transfer is the most basic action in all chemical reactions of the body. Using the PER 2000 the spin of the electron is increased, usually lasting about four days. In turn, this restores or replenishes the transmembrane potential of the cell – 'recharging the batteries' inside of you.

Healthy cells according to Nobel Prize winner Otto Warburg have cell transmembrane potential (TMP) voltages of negative 70 to 90 mV (millivolts). Due to the constant stresses of modern life and a toxic environment, cell voltage tends to drop as we age or get sick. As the voltage drops, the cell is unable to maintain a healthy environment for itself. If the electrical charge of the cell drops to negative 50 mV a person may experience chronic fatigue and under that a lower Rouleaux index. At roughly negative 18 mV conditions are ideal for cancer to develop. It takes a lot of energy to maintain negative 70 to 90 mV.

Rustem Roy, in *Science of Whole Person Healing*, reports it is known that damaged or diseased cells present an abnormally low TMP, about 80 percent lower than healthy cells.

This form of therapy may improve a variety of vital bodily functions: oxygen carrying capacity, assimilation of nutrients, manufacture of enzymes, metabolic waste removal, reduction of free radicals, tissue regeneration, normalisation of the membrane potential of diseased cells, changes in intracellular and extracellular ion concentration, increase in collagen and glycosaminoglycan syntheses, and healing and pain reduction.

The Theracell 100 Machine from Germany and PER 2000 from the USA are used to treat pain and are also being researched for:

- muscle strain
- ligament sprains
- cartilage tears
- joint and nerve inflammation
- pulled muscles
- back strain
- tennis elbow
- golfers elbow

- slipped disc
- herniated disc
- torn anterior cruciate ligament (knee)
- whiplash
- shin splints
- plantar fascitis (runner's knee)
- alzheimer's disease
- arthritis
- cerebral palsy
- chronic fatigue
- chronic fibromyalgia
- chronic pain
- cranial nerve dysfunction
- degenerative disc disease
- multiple sclerosis
- parkinson's disease
- peripheral neuropathy
- sports injuries
- stroke impairment
- temporomandibular joint dysfunction

Unlike TENS, no electrical current is used. The E Pulse 8000 is also being used, a technology that is known as Nuclear Magnetic Resonance (NMR) which is also a term being used for PEMF devices.

Note: This therapy is not used on individuals with implanted medical devices such as aneurysm clips in the brain, heart pacemakers or cochlear (inner ear) implants. Pregnancy, epilepsy and joint implants may also be conditions not eligible for NIIT treatment.

Radiowave Therapy

Compelling research has come to light regarding the efficacy of precision-focused RF energy. An earlier review was conducted for all work done up to 1999, but the treatment methods and technology are constantly being improved.

The three modalities that are currently used for cancer treatment are: surgery, radiation (ionizing), and chemotherapy. As the overall contribution of chemotherapy (curative and adjuvant cytotoxic) to five-year survival in adults was estimated to be 2.3 percent in Australia and 2.1 percent in the United States[13] a fourth modality (the scientific term is hyperthermia) using ultra-high-frequency (UHF) radiowaves as an adjunct is now being suggested.

As this treatment uses precision RF energy no damage is done to surrounding healthy tissue.

This radiowave therapy targets all cancers, and irrefutable proof on the success of hyperthermia treatment combined with radiation has been reported for the following nine tumor areas:

- head and neck
- GBM
- breast
- rectum
- melanoma
- bladder
- oesophagus
- cervix
- sarcomas

In advanced high-risk prostatic cancer, hyperthermia is feasible and well tolerated.[14]

In Europe this therapy is considered safe and has been used for over 20 years at the Heinrich Heine University in Germany. Dr Rudiger Wessalouski has been treating children over 20 years. Dusseldorf University combines hypothermia with chemotherapy under MRI combination for observation.

Dr Jacobi van der Zee PhD of the Daniel den Hoed Cancer Centre in Rotterdam and other doctors in the USA and Japan have worked together on clinical trials. Van der Zee demonstrated that the use of UHF plus low-dose radiation is a considerable improvement on conventional therapies without the often, devastating side effects.[15] Van der Zee has been working in this area for almost thirty years with her research being backed by the Dutch government as well as the Dutch Cancer Council.

Beginning in early 2009, the Dutch government reimburses citizens for hyperthermia therapy, the equivalent in Australia of a rebate (Medicare) from the federal government. This process, which has taken 20 years, acknowledges the work of Dr van der Zee and her colleagues.

Dr Sergio Maluta, head of the Radiation Oncology Department at the Azienda Ospedaliera Istituti Ospitalieri Di Verona, Italy is currently in discussions with the Italian government regarding rebates for the Italian people.

Currently the European Society for Hyperthermic Oncology (ESHO) is conducting a clinical trial across three countries on the best combination for the treatment of cancer using this fourth modality. The trials are being conducted in clinics in: Verona in Italy, Munich, Berlin and Erlangen in Germany, and Rotterdam in the Netherlands. The 29th Annual Meeting of the ESHO was held in Italy in 2014.

Dr Nisar Syed, director of Radiation Oncology, and Dr Ajmel Puthawala of Long Beach Memorial Hospital in Los Angeles have nearly 30 years' experience using this therapy.

Formerly of the United Kingdom and having practised in Western Australia, Dr John Holt conducted research and treatment for over 30 years. He became intrigued when his father, who was in his thirties at the time, was successfully treated for cancer of the eye in Paris by Dr Andre Denier who used hyperthermia treatment. Holt's father had the eyeball removed in his teenage years but the cancer continued to grow. After Denier's therapy he lived into his eighties.

Holt was led to investigate further treatments in regard to electrical energy in the quest to cure cancer. Working with UHF 434 MHz radiowaves, Holt is known for his additional use of a glucose-blocking agent now being researched in Ireland and India.

Holt examined the work of Dr Otto Warburg, who in 1920 found that a tumor has hardly any oxygen. In 1931 the Nobel Prize in Physiology or Medicine was awarded to Warburg, who first discovered that cancer cells have a fundamentally different energy metabolism compared to healthy cells. Nominated an unprecedented three times for the Nobel Prize for three separate achievements, Warburg won the Nobel Prize for his 'discovery of the nature and mode of action of the respiratory enzyme'. When the respiration process of cells goes wrong, they can become cancerous: cancer cells function best in the absence of oxygen, in effect, living on fermentation rather than respiration. According to Warburg, cancer should be interpreted as a mitochondrial dysfunction.

The theories of Warburg have in recent times gained more attention in view of findings linking the impairment of mitochondria with a breakdown in normal cell apoptotic (mechanism that allows cells to self-destruct when stimulated by the appropriate trigger) processes and tumor growth.

Of particular interest, Holt observed differences in the power spectrum of the radiowave waveform emitted by cancer patient's bodies during radiowave treatment, compared to the spectrum of people without cancer.

Holt argued that radiowaves at the specific frequency of 434MHz have a non-thermal (biological) effect on the physiology of cancer cells, namely increased cell division or some changes in the electrochemistry of cells evidenced by resonance effects.

Holt also postulated that 434 MHz radiowaves increase the rate of cell division and that this will result in more cancer cells being starved of energy following the administration of GMI – injection of a compound referred to as 'glycolytic metabolic inhibitors' – to disrupt the metabolism of cancer cells prior to exposure to radiowaves.

Since Holt's retirement the non-profit privately funded Radiowave Therapy Research Institute (RTRI) in Claremont, Australia, has taken over his treatment methods and is treating patients and collating the research. IT Sligo, Charles River Laboratories (CRL), John Hopkins School of Medicine, Curtin University, Radiowave Therapy Clinic, and Dublin Institute of Technology are advising, involved with and/or carrying out radiowave therapy cancer research with RTRI.

Oncothermia

Hyperthermia is the artificial method of inducing heat from external sources to the human body utilizing microwaves, EMF, radio antennas, infrared etc., thereby increasing the temperature of a specific part of the body, such as the tumor, in the aim to kill the maximum number of cancer cells. Oncothermia does not rely on heat alone as a principle of treatment.

The Oncothermia principle was originally developed in Scotland with the first research published by professor Andras Szasz, Department of Biotechnics at St Istvan University, Hungary. The principles are based on hyperthermia however, beside the absolute increase in temperature, the aim is especially the direct electric field energy absorption in the extracellular liquid and destroying the membrane of the cancer cells.

This method transfers energy using the principle of capacitive coupling. An electric field, produced by two active electrodes passes through the patient's body. The electric field tends to move through the pathways with the lowest impedance – through the malignant tissue (tumor).

The Oncothermia treatment induces an electromagnetic field on the conductivity of current passing the near-membrane electrolytes of the cancer cell. Cancer cells during the time they have been exposed to the field begin to heat and then die. As the flow of current is restricted by the number of cancer cells being affected temperature is developed.

Dr Carl Munoz-Ferrada explains that with the dosimetry utilized in hyperthermia, the margin between cancerous cells and good cells is no more than 2°C: if the good cells are hit about 44°C they begin to be killed but cancer cells do not have the capability to withstand temperatures above 42°C. The treatment has to be very precise: hyperthermia can bring an extra supply of blood containing glucose and other metabolites that can help the tumor grow instead of minimizing it. Also the higher blood-flow increases the risk of dissemination of malignant cells.

Oncothermia does not produce any secondary effects and can be delivered with traditional therapies such as Linac-radiotherapy and chemotherapy, or, as a stand-alone therapy for areas where these two other traditional therapies cannot reach or it is too risky to use them.

This treatment is performed in Austria, Belgium, Canada, China, Denmark, Germany, Greece, Hungary, Israel, Italy, Jordan, Romania, Russia, South Korea, The Netherlands, Turkey and Ukraine.

A partnership has been set up between Gammasonics Institute for Medical Research, Canada Bay Medical Centre and Southern Radiology for the setting up of treatment clinics across Australia.

The private Jenny Barlow Oncothermia Clinic at the Prince of Wales Hospital in Sydney opened in November 2012.

Therabionic Therapy

American and Brazilian cancer researchers have succeeded in stabilizing and shrinking inoperable liver tumors with RF radiation that is no more powerful than that emitted by a typical mobile phone. Boris Pasche, director of the Division of Hematology and Oncology at the University of Alabama School of Medicine in Birmingham and Frederico Costa, director of clinical research at the Brazilian Institute for Research on Cancer in São Paulo observed significant tumor shrinkage in 10 percent of patients. Costa points out that this is five times the success rate of the best available chemotherapeutic drug – Sorafenib – and that 'there are essentially no side effects'.

Liver cancer is the second most frequent cause of cancer mortality among men worldwide. For women, it is the sixth leading cause of cancer death.

This new therapy called TheraBionic could revolutionize the treatment of liver cancer. Patients with liver tumors, hepatocellular carcinoma (HCC) that cannot be completely removed during surgery, have a very poor prognosis. Average survival time is just 3–6 months. While the median overall survival of the 41 patients in Costa and Pasche's treatment group was only somewhat longer (6.7 months), eight of their patients had a remarkable response. Six of the eight went on to live for more than two years – four of them for at least three years. Notably, five of the six long-term survivors had tumors that were actively growing when they began receiving RF therapy. One of these five, a 76-year old woman, was still alive and being treated close to five years later.

Four (9.8 percent) of Costa and Pasche's 41 patients with terminal liver cancer saw the size of their tumors decrease by at least 30 percent. By comparison, in a similar trial using the drug Sorafenib, only three of 137 patients (2 percent) showed the same level of tumor response. In all, eight of the patients receiving RF therapy either saw their tumors shrink or they survived for longer than two years, or both.

The RF therapy also helped many of the patients who were in pain. Of the 11 patients reporting pain before entering the trial, five said that it completely disappeared and two said that it decreased soon after treatment began.

There was no change for two others – two complained that there was more pain after treatment.

One clear inference from the trial is that some patients were much more responsive to RF therapy than others. The reasons why are unknown.

Pasche explained that all sorts of different people fared better, without any obvious traits in common. 'Both men and women, Caucasian and non-Caucasian, patients with hepatitis B, hepatitis C or no hepatitis infection responded to the therapy,' he said.

Even though Pasche and Costa don't have a mechanism in hand to explain how the radiation can control the growth of the tumors, they state that their 'novel therapeutic approach does not depend on temperature changes within the tumor'.

TheraBionic treatment uses a device that looks like a spatula connected to a box slightly larger than a mobile phone. The spatula is a stainless steel antenna that transmits 27.12 MHz amplitude modulated (AM) radiation generated by an amplifier inside the box. Patients put the antenna in their mouths for one hour, three times a day. Treatment can be done at home and does not require hospitalization.

The maximum SAR is less than 2 W/Kg, averaged over 10g of tissue in the mouth near the antenna. It is much, much lower inside the tumor. Pasche estimates that the dose to the cancer cells is 100 to 1,000 times lower than that from a cell phone. 'When you take the mouthpiece and put it in your mouth, the body becomes an antenna – the whole body receives a tiny but fairly homogeneous amount of RF,' he states.

The key to the new therapy appears to be a cocktail of frequencies riding on the 27 MHz signal. Over the course of the one-hour treatment, the RF generator runs through 194 different modulations, beginning with 410 Hz and rising to 21 kHz. Each one lasts three seconds. At the end of the cycle, the sequence repeats itself.

The 194 specific frequencies for liver cancer were identified using biofeed-back techniques, which consist of measuring variations in skin electrical resistance, pulse-amplitude and blood pressure. In the process, the international team identified other 'tumor-specific frequencies', including those for treating brain, breast, ovarian and prostate cancers.

'We believe this treatment has great potential and will be explored for other types of cancer,' Costa said. He described how one of his patients with breast cancer, metastatic to the adrenal gland and bone, had a 'complete response' after an 11-month treatment. The woman received a different set of frequencies, though they were in the same range (100 Hz to 21 kHz) as those used for liver tumors.

The relative efficacy of the 194 HCC frequencies will be tested in an upcoming study. This trial, which will be run in Brazil and the USA will include 272 patients, randomly assigned to one of two treatment groups: one will get TheraBionic signals and the other randomly chosen frequencies. Costa and James Posey of the University of Alabama are co-principal investigators of the new study. If these trials are successful, the next step would be to obtain USA FDA approval for widespread use of TheraBionic therapy, which has already been discussed with the FDA, with the protocol being revized and approved by the agency.

In addition Pasche is running both cellular and animal studies in his lab at the University of Alabama, using exposure systems designed by the University's Department of Radiation Oncology and Kuster's group in Zurich.

Costa and Pasche's new findings were published by the *British Journal of Cancer*.[16]

TTF Therapy

In May 2011 the FDA cleared Novocure's NovoTTF first-of-a-kind treatment device specifically for a tumor type known as glioblastoma, the most aggressive form of brain cancer. This fourth approach fights brain tumors using electrical energy fields.

The NovoTTF-100A is a non-invasive portable device for continuous use through the day consisting of 4 sets of insulated electrodes attached to an electronic box. The electrical current is sent from the device to the electrodes which are attached to the patient's shaved head. The 3 kilogram device is carried by the patient in a small bag. NovoCure uses 100–200 kHz electric fields – the company calls them tumor treating fields or TTFields – to stunt the growth of cancer cells, either by slowing down their proliferation or by killing them off entirely.

The device creates a low intensity, alternating electric field within the tumor that exerts physical forces on electrically charged cellular components, preventing the normal mitotic process and causing cancer cell death prior to division – cancer cells divide and multiply rapidly in the brain carrying specific electrically charged elements that play a role during the cell division process.

Due to the unique shape of cancer cells, when they are multiplying, TTFields cause the building blocks of these cells to pile up in such a way that the cells physically break apart. In addition, cancer cells also contain miniature building blocks that move essential parts of the cells from place to place during division. TTFields cause these building blocks to fall apart since they have a special type of electric charge. As a result of these two effects, preliminary study data indicate that cancer tumor growth is slowed and may even reverse after continuous exposure to TTFields.

The FDA approval was based on data from a randomized pivotal trial of 237 patients with glioblastoma tumors that had recurred or progressed despite previous surgical, radiation and chemotherapy treatments. Patients treated with the NovoTTF alone achieved a comparable overall survival time to patients treated with the physician's choice of the best chemotherapy, but had fewer side effects, and reported improved quality of life scores. Results from a pilot study of the device suggest that the investigational treatment may increase the length of time before disease progression and increase median overall survival for newly diagnosed GBM patients. Novocure is sponsoring an ongoing pivotal trial of the NovoTTF for patients with newly diagnosed glioblastoma tumors.

Unlike chemotherapy or radiation, based on the limited clinical results to date, the NovoTTF-100A does not appear to have significant side effects. Most patients have experienced skin irritation beneath the electrodes. No device-related serious adverse events were observed in over 400 patient-months of cumulative exposure to NovoTTF-100A treatment.

The NovoTTF-100A device was invented by emeritus professor Yoram Palti MD at the Technion – Israel Institute of Technology, the leading Israeli biomedical research institution. Novocure currently has US and European marketing approvals for the NovoTTF-100A.[17]

Implanting Electrodes

In a move that gives cautious hope to the millions of people suffering some form of paralysis, in May 2011 a research team from University of California, Los Angeles (UCLA), Caltech and the University of Louisville has given a man, rendered paralyzed from the chest down after a hit-and-run accident in 2006, the ability to stand and take his first tentative steps in four years.

Neuroscientists implanted 16 electrodes in his spine and sent electrical impulses to his lower spinal cord, mimicking the signals normally sent by the brain to initiate movement. Researchers are hopeful that their work could one day provide some individuals suffering spinal cord injuries with the ability to stand independently, maintain balance and take effective steps through the use of a portable stimulation unit and the assistance of a walker. Additionally, the researchers believe the approach could potentially also help in the treatment of stroke, Parkinson's and other disorders affecting motor function.

The work was funded by the National Institutes of Health and the Christopher & Dana Reeve Foundation.[18]

NanoKnife

Cancer Treatment Centers of America state NanoKnife® provides a minimally invasive option for patients with inoperable or difficult-to-reach tumors, including tumors located near critical structures and major blood vessels in the body. Instead of using microwave energy, extreme heat or extreme cold, the NanoKnife System uses electrical currents to treat tumors.

While the patient is under general anesthesia, the interventional radiologist carefully guides up to six thin needles (electrodes) into the patient's body and strategically places them around the tumor. Then, the NanoKnife System sends electrical pulses or currents between each set of needles to puncture permanent nanometer-sized holes into the tumor. This process, called irreversible electroporation (IRE), causes the cancer cells to be unbalanced and triggers a cell 'suicide', thereby destroying the tumor.

The electrical pulses are contained between the electrodes, minimizing damage to surrounding healthy cell tissue, blood vessels and other important structures. After the tumor is destroyed, the body naturally rids itself of the dead cells, which are replaced with healthy cells.

The procedure lasts from two to four hours. After the procedure, the patient is hospitalized overnight for observation and typically discharged the following day. The patient is also given antibiotics before and after the procedure to prevent infection.

Potential benefits of NanoKnife include:

- no open incisions
- less damage to healthy tissue
- minimal post-operative pain
- fewer side effects
- short hospital stay
- quick post-operative recovery
- ability to repeat the procedure if new tumors develop

NanoKnife may be a treatment option for patients who are not candidates for conventional treatments or if other treatments were not effective. Patients with a cardiac pacemaker, abnormal heartbeat or nerve stimulators are not eligible for this procedure.

Even though this is a minimally invasive technique as opposed to a non-invasive technique, it is included to show that the worlds of invasive and non-invasive ways of treating people are becoming closer. Another example is Proton Beam Therapy, an advance over traditional radiotherapy because the radiation beam is targeted only to the tumor, better sparing surrounding healthy tissue from harm.

LIGHT AS ENERGY

Natural EMF and sunlight is composed of a variety of energies that are transmitted to Earth in the form of electromagnetic waves. Light is a nutrient that streams from the Sun, flowing through our eyes and triggering hormone production, influencing the complex bio-system which ultimately affects our whole being. Natural light is a non-invasive powerful tool, the basic component from which all life originates, develops, heals and evolves. We cannot survive without light energy. When bare skin is exposed to natural sunlight – ultraviolet B (UVB) – the body makes vitamin D.

With his pioneering suggestion to look into the role of 'transients' in the breast cancer cluster at San Diego, as far back as 1990, Cedric Garland, along with his brother Frank Garland, Edward Gorham and Jeffrey Young, was pivotal in bringing attention to vitamin D playing a role in reducing breast cancer risk. Breast cancer was one of the first cancers identified as having protection from vitamin D.

In 2012 at Georgetown University Medical Center (GUMC) in Washington DC, another link was found between high vitamin D intake and a reduced risk of breast cancer. A study with mice revealed that high doses of vitamin D are linked to a 50 percent reduction in tumor cases and a 75 percent reduction in overall cancer growth among those who already have the disease.[19]

The rate of breast cancer appears to decrease by approximately 30 percent when vitamin D levels in the blood are greater than 100 nmol/L (40 ng/ml) compared to lower levels of 50 nmol/L (20 ng/ml).

The Vitamin D Council states low vitamin D levels impair DNA repair mechanisms, and having optimal levels of vitamin D better manages calcium in the blood, bones and gut, and aids in cell communication. Individuals are classed as vitamin D deficient at 50 nmol/L (20 ng/ml) which can be monitored by a blood test for 25(OH)D levels. The Vitamin D Council recommends levels between 125-200 nmol/L (50-80 ng/ml) though there is debate worldwide about optimum levels.

The Vitamin D Council reports the body can produce 10,000 to 25,000 IU of vitamin D in less than the time it takes the skin to turn pink. The paler the skin type – roughly only 15 minutes required each day – the more easily the skin can produce vitamin D. This also prevents burning the skin. Dark skin types do not burn so easily and the darker the skin type the longer one has to stay exposed to sunlight. The more skin that is exposed, the more Vitamin D one can produce. If one's shadow is smaller than one is tall, the individual is making vitamin D. This occurs closer to the middle of the day. If one's shadow is longer than one is tall then one is not making much vitamin D. Sunscreens and sunblocks usually block vitamin D production.

Vitamin D3 is actually a hormone providing information to the DNA in every cell in the body and estimated to control at least 1,000 genes by either turning them on or turning them off. The Vitamin D Council states a lack of vitamin D has been linked to conditions such as cancer, asthma, type 2 diabetes, high blood pressure, depression, Alzheimer's, and autoimmune diseases like multiple sclerosis, Crohn's and type 1 diabetes.

The Vitamin D Council states previous research has linked low levels of vitamin D with increasing one's risk of stroke and a variety of cardiovascular events and mortality. In December 2013 a study from China found that vitamin D levels predict short-term disability outcomes and death in those who suffered acute ischemic stroke (AIS), the most common type of stroke. Furthermore, the researchers found that low vitamin D levels were associated with increased risk of death after stroke and disability after stroke.[20]

Pregnant women are encouraged to have optimum levels and another area of research is whether low levels of vitamin D for mother and child are a co-factor in the development of autism.

Photobiologist Dr John Ott states there are strong indications that UV light through the eyes stimulates the immune system. Near UV (UVA 320–380 nm) is responsible for the tanning response. Mid UV (UVB 290–320 nm) seems to activate the synthesis of vitamin D and the absorption of calcium and other minerals. Far UV (UVC 100–290 nm) – mostly filtered out by the Earth's ozone layer – is germicidal, killing bacteria, viruses and other infectious agents.[21]

UV light has been shown to:

- activate the synthesis of vitamin D
- lower blood pressure
- increase the efficiency of the heart
- improve electrocardiogram (ECG) readings and blood profiles of individuals with atherosclerosis (hardening of the arteries)

- reduce cholesterol
- assist in weight loss
- effective treatment for psoriasis and many other diseases
- increase the level of sex hormones
- activate an important skin hormone – solitrol.[22]

It is the discovery that lack of light is the cause of Seasonal Affective Disorder (SAD) that helped propel light therapy technologies. SAD happens in most countries of the world where the winter brings short daylight hours and long dark evenings. Light treatment also known as phototherapy is now used extensively throughout the world in psychiatric hospitals and clinics.

The Danish physician Niels Ryberg Finsen founded modern light therapy over 100 years ago and in 1903 he was awarded the Nobel Prize in Medicine for his achievements with light therapy. Finsen created the first device to generate technically synthesized sunlight and achieved outstanding results in the treatment of patients suffering from a special type of skin tuberculosis. He also used red light in the treatment of smallpox lesions.

Today it is known that the human organism transforms light into electrochemical energy, activating a chain of biochemical reactions with cells, stimulating metabolism and reinforcing the immune response of the entire body. Treating a patient with light adds energy to the target tissue, boosting energy to the cells to accelerate healing.

What we perceive as light is a form of energy that behaves like a wave and also as a stream of particles called photons. Each photon gyrates and bounces at a unique frequency and exhibits electrical and magnetic properties.

Cells absorb photons and transform their energy into ATP, the energy molecule of nearly all living creatures. The resulting ATP is then used to power metabolic processes, synthesize DNA, RNA, proteins, enzymes, and other products needed to repair or regenerate cell components, foster mitosis or cell proliferation and restore homeostasis.

The first systematic research into the role of light in living processes was done by Russian scientist Alexander Gurwitsch who established as a conclusive hypothesis that every living cell emits light, though at a very weak level.

With Fritz-Albert Popp's photomultiplier machine, it was possible to prove beyond any doubt that low-level light emissions are a common property of all living cells. Popp found biophotons (information particles) control the body's metabolism and processes. Biophotons are photons emitted spontaneously by all living systems. The use of photo emission is able to show clear distinctions appear between healthy cells and cancer cells in the coherence-quality differences of their emitted light. The better the transmission of information in coherent light, the better the cell.

When researchers at the Max Planck Institute in Germany looked at human DNA down to the subatomic level, all they encountered was light – coherent light. Physicist David Bohm states that all matter is frozen light.

Sunlight, at an effective temperature of 5,780 kelvins, is composed of nearly thermal-spectrum radiation that is slightly more than half infrared. At zenith, sunlight provides an irradiance of just over 1 kilowatts per square meter at sea level. Of this energy, 527 watts is infrared radiation, 445 watts is visible light, and 32 watts is ultraviolet radiation.

Only a tiny percent of the electromagnetic spectrum is believed to be perceived by the human eye. The visible portion of the electromagnetic spectrum from the most beautiful violet to the most intense red is essential for human life. The visible wavelengths of violet, indigo, blue, green, yellow, orange and red are from the shortest to the longest. When we see color, the photoreceptor cells of the retina in our eyes converts the color into electrical impulses. These impulses travel to the brain and trigger reactions in the endocrine – hormone release – system.

Light comes in different colors, with each color corresponding to waves with different wavelengths. Different colors of light carry differing amounts of energy: high frequency, short wavelength purple light carries the most energy and low frequency, long wavelength red light carries the least energy.

Waves with wavelengths slightly shorter than purple light, and thus have slightly higher frequencies and higher energy levels, are called ultraviolet (UV) – 'beyond violet' – which humans cannot see. Likewise, just beyond the other end of the visible spectrum are waves with wavelengths slightly longer than red light waves. These waves, which have even lower frequencies and carry somewhat less energy than red light, are called infrared (IR) – 'below red'.

APPROXIMATE GUIDE TO THE WAVELENGTHS AND FREQUENCIES		
	WAVELENGTH	FREQUENCY
IR	1mm–700 nm	300–430 THz
Red	700–635 nm	430–480 THz
Orange	635–590 nm	480–510 THz
Yellow	590–560 nm	510–540 THz
Green	560–490 nm	540–610 THz
Blue	490–450 nm	610–670 THz
Indigo	450–425 nm	670–700 THz
Violet	425–380 nm	700–750 THz
UV	380–10 nm	750 THz – 30 PHz

LIGHT TREATMENTS

PHOTOBIOMODULATION

Photobiomodulation – also known as low-level (or 'cold') laser therapy (LLLT) – is a non-invasive clinical application of light and its action mechanisms on cellular and molecular levels have been studied for over 30 years. Usually produced by low to mid-power lasers, more recently Light Emitting Diodes (LEDs) are used: the coherent and incoherent light with the same wavelength, intensity and dose providing the same biological response.

Tiina Karu PhD, of the Institute of Laser and Information Technologies of Russian Academy of Sciences, Moscow, Russian Federation states in *Is it Time to Consider Photobiomodulation as a Drug Equivalent?*:

> The rather old suggestion the photoacceptor for photobiomodulation effects is cytochrome c oxidase has been confirmed by now. The new data support the old conclusion that photobiomodulation is more pronounced in ill or otherwise stressed cells, as compared with healthy cells with plenty of oxygen available. The terminal enzyme of the mitochondrial respiratory chain and its electronic excitation by light with proper parameters causes retrograde light-sensitive cellular signaling events to transport the light signal from mitochondria to the nucleus to cause gene expression. The gene expression events caused by irradiation are confirmed and have been studied in more detail in recent years.

In the 1930s, Emmitt Knott and Virgil Hancock pioneered the idea of using a converted Hanovia water-cooled UV lamp for the purpose of irradiating blood. Bacterially infected blood was cleaned by this process and then returned to the body. In St Petersburg, professor Kira Samoilova, head of Photobiology at the Russian Academy of Sciences claims success in treating lung, intestinal and breast cancers, stomach ulcers and more. In the treatment about five percent of the blood in the body is passed through the irradiating device once or twice a day for as long as necessary.

Intranasal Light Therapy

Today LLLT has built up a substantial body of evidence to support the indication that it is able to achieve red blood cell (RBC) disaggregation, lower viscosity and hence better blood circulation. The improved blood circulation is achieved from the method of illuminating the blood – blood irradiation.

Blood is fundamental to the survival and propagation of human life and the body cannot function well without a strong circulatory system. Intranasal Light Therapy is now being used to assist in stimulating the body to re-establish its natural internal balance – homeostasis.

All of the blood passes through the nasal blood vessels every minute and close to the surface. Intranasal Light Therapy is non-invasive blood irradiation delivering low level light into the vascular rich capillary bed in the nasal cavity. The vascular walls in the nasal cavity region are particularly thin and sensitive, making them highly receptive to any biostimulation. Irradiation of these surface blood vessels with the right frequency of pure red light positively affects the blood cells by restoring their electrical charge. Changes in the RBC aggregation (Rouleaux Index) have been observed in small blood samples taken before and after each preset session under a microscope.

INFRARED

Discovered by astronomer William Herschel in 1800, IR light is slightly more than half of the total energy from the Sun. IR light is absorbed by human tissue in the same way plants feed on the Sun's energy during photosynthesis. IR energy is also one of the ways in which our cells communicate with each other – biological induction. Today near-infrared (0.76–1.56 microns), mid-infrared (1.5–4 microns) and far-infrared (4–1000 microns) applications are being used in industrial, scientific and medical applications.

The far-infrared (FIR) rays are the invisible rays of natural sunlight that have the longest wavelength. The most beneficial found to be the waves between 6 and 14 microns, with the best absorption rate at 9.4 microns. Humans cannot see infrared light but they can feel it. We continuously radiate IR energy through the surface of the skin at between 3 and 50 microns with most of its output hovering around 9.4 microns.

All living organisms including humans emit and absorb IR energy. A young vital body can send out a lot of IR power as opposed to an individual in ill health who loses much of their ability to emit IR waves. Our palms emit FIR energy between 8 and 14 microns and it is believed that the 'power' of the palms of Qigong masters is the intensity of their FIR energy. It is believed FIR rays set up a resonance in the body – the waves work by vibrating at the same rate of the body. There is evidence that IR radiation from the hands of Qigong practitioners can increase cell growth, DNA and protein synthesis, and cell respiration. (There is also evidence that living systems emit microwaves.)[23]

FIR therapy, which penetrates into the human body, is used for the treatment of a wide variety of health problems. Used as a deliberate heating source, the heat from IR light penetrates the skin deeper and is seen to be more efficient than other heating methods.

IR therapy can gently raise the body core temperature by 3°C and activate major bodily functions, relieving pain, reducing inflammation, decrease muscle spasms and increase blood circulation. By increasing circulation to the area of sporting injuries this therapy increases transport of the materials essential for rebuilding damaged tissue, thereby reducing recovery time. IR light is reported to be able to regenerate cells 200 to 400 times faster than the process normally takes.

In general, IR light therapy is thought to promote a strong immune system and cardiovascular system, increasing blood circulation without straining the heart. It is believed IR light rays stimulate killer T-cells, white blood cell and oxygen levels in the blood and help to boost collagen production while enhancing stem cell circulation. It can be helpful in treating conditions characterized by pain and inflammation including:

- arthritis
- back pain
- bursitis
- carpal tunnel syndrome
- fibromyalgia
- muscle sprains and strains
- neck pain
- rheumatoid arthritis
- sciatica
- temporomandibular joint pain
- tendonitis
- wounds

Red and near-infrared have beneficial effects on cells by 'kick-starting' them into immediately creating more ATP (cellular energy) and increasing DNA and RNA activity. Injured cells need the extra ATP to repair themselves. About 35 percent of the energy in this range is absorbed by a specific 'proton pump' (cytochrome c oxidase, CCO, 'complex IV') in mitochondria. The light at specific wavelengths 'kick-start' the CCO pump into producing more cellular energy: ATP. The key is in delivery of correct wavelengths under controlled dosage.

IR is used in many different forms. For example, medical grade IR is used for facial rejuvenation and the MIRoTEC wrap uses space blanket technology to reflect back body heat and stimulate the lymphatic system. IR is also used in mild hyperthermia – IR saunas, domes and arches.

The balance between absorbed and emitted IR radiation also has a critical effect on Earth's climate.

Onnetsu Ki wand

The Onnetsu Ki wand is based on the Japanese traditional concept that degenerated, diseased or inactive cells or tissues are lacking energy (or heat) and are therefore 'cold'. This coldness shows up on the surface of skin above. The wand finds not only these damaged spots deep inside the body but also provides the healing energy of FIR, rejuvenating cells and promoting blood circulation and Ki flow.

By moving the Onnetsu Ki over the body, the patient experiences some areas as 'hot' because the skin there is cold and the sensation manifests as 'hot'. In the case of cancer, cells are extremely cold and the patient may even feel pain. By applying the wand on these areas repeatedly, the FIR energy goes deep inside the body (4–5 inches deep) giving FIR energy to these cells and tissues. When the heat reaches and warms up the cells, those areas no longer feel hot and healing starts.

HEALS technology

In the early 1990s, Quantum Devices Inc teamed with the Wisconsin Center for Space Automation and Robotics – a NASA-sponsored research centre at the University of Wisconsin-Madison – to develop Astroculture 3, a plant growth chamber using near IR High Emissivity Aluminiferous Luminescent Substrate (HEALS) technology for plant growth experiments on shuttle missions. Over the years, Quantum Devices Inc has worked to develop HEALS technology for use in medical fields, specifically with pediatric brain tumors and hard-to-heal wounds such as diabetic skin ulcers and serious burns.

In a two-year clinical trial, cancer patients undergoing bone marrow or stem cell transplants were given HEALS – a far red/near IR LED treatment – to treat oral mucositis, a common and extremely painful side effects of chemotherapy and radiation treatment. This technology successfully reduced the painful side effects in bone marrow and stem cell transplant patients.

The WARP 75 light delivery system (one of the many devices using HEALS technology) uses HEALS technology to provide intense light energy: the equivalent light energy of 12 Suns from each of the 288 LED chips. (The LED – about the size of a grain of salt – produces 12 times more radiant energy than the Sun in the same bandwidth). HEALS technology allows LED – light sources releasing energy in the form of photons – chips to function at their maximum irradiancy without emitting heat.

HEALS technology activates light-sensitive, tumor-treating drugs that completely destroy cancer cells while leaving the surrounding tissue virtually untouched. Research is continuing for the treatment of brain injuries, strokes, bone atrophy, MS, Parkinson's disease, Alzheimer's disease, pressure sores, wound healing, depression and degenerative retina/eye disorders.[24]

HEALS technology has won numerous accolades, including the Space Technology Hall of Fame award, the Marshall Space Flight Center Hallmark of Success award, the Wisconsin Governor's New Product Award, and the prestigious Tibbetts Award as an SBIR success story.

QUANTUM THERAPY

Quantum Therapy has been used to treat the following conditions for nearly 30 years:

- sports traumas:stretchings, bruises, damages of sheaves, joints, muscles, bones
- cardiovascular and nervous diseases, relaxation, stress
- bronchial-pulmonary diseases, especially when combined with nebulizing therapy for acute, chronic pains
- diseases of the digestive, urogenital systems
- cosmetology

Introscan

The Introscan, a Quantum Therapy physiotherapy unit, is easy to use and is driven by its software package that can be loaded onto any Windows based computer. On selecting the health issue, the software guides the individual through the placement of the unit on each of the relevant treatment areas. The high efficiency of the Introscan device is achieved by using a combination of visible spectrum light, laser IR and UV, incorporating those signals with different types of modulated frequencies on acupuncture points that affect specific organs and systems.

Acupuncture points are energetic communication gateways and highly responsive to light. Gerber states acupuncture points – acupoints – can be located on the skin via their characteristic of low electrical resistance, i.e., high conductivity, which is consistent with their role as portals of energy entry into the body. He also reports that electrographic scans of the body demonstrate that acupuncture points glow brightly when their associated meridian is out of balance, thus allowing an alternative method of disease detection. According to acupuncture researcher Ion Dumitrescu of Romania the electrodermal points are electrical pores – concerning two-way energy exchange between the body and the environment.

Conditions that are being treated include:

- acne
- acute and chronic bronchial pneumonia
- algomenorrhea, pelvic pain, endometriosis
- angina, exacerbation of chronic tonsillitis
- areas of the spine, osteochondrosis, spondylosis deformans, spondylarthrosis
- atherosclerosis (aka arteriosclerotic vascular disease or ASVD), obliterating endarteritis
- bronchial asthma
- burns and frostbite (aka congelatio)
- cellulitis
- cervical erosion
- chronic non-specific colitis, constipation
- chronic pancreatitis, acute stage
- cystitis
- duodenum diseases, duodenal ulcer, duodenitis, cicatricial changes in the duodenum
- eczema, neurodermatitis, toxicoderma, psoriasis
- enuresis, dysuria associated with the bladder and urethra
- epilepsy
- finger joints
- fungal nail plates (aka onychomycosis)
- gallbladder diseases and bile duct diseases
- gastroenterology (children)
- haemorrhoids
- hypertension
- inflammatory diseases with signs of suppuration
- irregular heartbeat
- ischemic heart disease
- liver disease, chronic hepatitis, fatty liver, cirrhosis of the liver
- non-invasive effects on blood
- otosclerosis, tinnitus, hearing loss

- periodontal disease
- pharyngitis, laryngotracheitis without stenosis of at most 1 degree
- post-operative scars
- prostate
- rejuvenation of the face and neck
- rhinitis (different clinical forms)
- sciatica
- sinusitis
- somatic stimulation for children over the age of three
- stomach diseases, chronic gastritis, stomach ulcer
- consequences of ischemia
- toe joints
- traumatic wounds – post-operative
- tympanoplasty, surgery replacing auditory ossicles in a plastic graft
- universal rehabilitation
- urethritis
- uterine fibroids, menstrual cycle functional disorders
- uterus and its appendages – inflammatory diseases, endometritis, salpingo-oophoritis
- venous insufficiency, varicose veins

POLARIZED LIGHT

Biophysicist Dr Marta Fenyö PhD, inventor of the Polychromatic Light System and Polarized Light and Bio-Stimulation, won the main award in 1985 at the World Exhibition of Young Inventors and also won a gold medal in Brussels in 1996. (Polychromatic means an emission of multiple wavelengths or colors. Polarized means light wavelengths are in parallel planes). This groundbreaking research revealed certain physical characteristics that are essential for the effectiveness of light therapy.

Fenyö has demonstrated unequivocally that polarized light is both bio-stimulatory and immuno-stimulatory. It has a direct and measurable effect at the cellular level. Bio-stimulation affects the membranes that cover each cell in our body. The result is accelerated healing.

The beneficial effect of polarized light has been proven in the tumor therapy of animals. Two groups of mice carried the Ehrlich Ascites tumor in their bodies. After treating the spleens of one group of mice with polarized light it was found that the growth of the tumor stopped. Later a small amount of the separated blood serum from the group of mice treated with polarized light was injected into the bodies of the untreated mice. The malignant process stopped in the untreated group as well. Consequently a material was produced in the blood serum of animals by polarized light that stopped the progression of the malignant process.

In another experiment conducted on mice, the daily treatment using polarized light resulted in total recovery in some cases and significantly extended the life of animals carrying a highly aggressive sarcoma where the experimental life expectancy was 28 days.

In another experiment with dying dogs Fenyo took some blood, irradiated it with polarized light and then reinjected the blood into the dogs. There was a dramatic reduction in tumor size, accompanied by a remarkable increase in alertness in the dogs.

BIOPTRON

A version of this technique uses a tool called the BIOPTRON which uses visible incoherent polarized (VIP) light, the most important aspect of the BIOPTRON device being the polarization of the emitted light. BIOPTRON state that the human organism transforms BIOPTRON light into electro-chemical energy that activates a chain of biochemical and enzymatic reactions. This device was created with a specific optical unit emitting light that is similar to the part of the electromagnetic spectrum produced naturally by the Sun but with *no UV radiation* (UVA or UBV). Sunburn is what we experience from UV. Once delivered to the tissues, the light energy promotes the process of bio-stimulation, stimulating diverse biological processes in organisms in a positive manner, enhancing bodily functions.

The BIOPTRON light is not at all similar to the Infrared Lamp. Whilst the spectrum of the BIOPTRON contains a fractional amount of near infrared, the wavelength of the light is much broader to incorporate the visible spectrum of 480–3400 nm. There are no thermal (heat) hazards with the BIOPTRON Light Therapy System. Uses of the Bioptron Light Therapy include:

- burns
- bed sores
- diabetic ulcers
- wound healing
- diseased gums
- collagen promotion, wrinkle smoothing
- improving vision and keeping the eye healthy
- asthma – oxygenating tissue and keeping the lungs healthy
- acne, eczema, certain types of psoriasis, chronic infantile skin diseases
- treating hair and skin problems on the skull (e.g. hair loss, dandruff, itching, or bleeding scalp)

- pain relief (e.g. gout, osteoarthritis, myositis, bursitis, rheumatoid arthritis, painful sports related injuries, sprains, tearing of a ligament, tense and rigid muscles, haemorrhoids, migraine, back pain, otitis media, tinnitus, bunions)
- acute pain in joints (e.g. tennis elbow, neck, shoulder & knee-joints)
- chronic rheumatic conditions (rheumatoid arthritis)
- build-up of lactic acid
- insomnia
- SAD and all forms of depression

This painless technology is also being used to treat burns from radiation and bombs. In Europe it is used as a medical device. There are no known side effects.

Fenyö has been researching this therapy's use in the treatment of cancer and her dream is to improve the quality of life of patients with cancer, as this treatment is harmless and painless.

Effective light therapy can enhance the immune system up to 50 percent. As this technology can help the immune system produce perfect cells and sustain it during therapy its use has significant implications for cancer treatment.[25]

Sensolite®

Fenyö and her team have advanced polarized light therapy even further. Not limited to a restricted surface of the body, Sensolite® therapy is whole body therapy with the beneficial effect of polarized light manifesting almost immediately on all cells of the body, exerting a stimulatory effect on metabolism, circulation, cell regeneration and cell function. Triggering healing mechanisms, the treatment has beneficial effects on the immune system, blood circulation and oxygen supply of the cells.

The treatment, using polarized light, significantly stimulates the activity of T-lymphocytes responsible for recognizing and defeating millions of faulty cells produced minute by minute in the human body that subsequently become responsible for serious illnesses and malignant deformations, thereby preventing more or less serious illnesses, as well as facilitating and accelerating the recovery from protracted illnesses.

This therapy is designed to mobilize the body's intrinsic defence mechanisms and Fenyö believes this can improve the health condition of patients by slowing down the progression of the malignant process. It has been long known that regeneration and cancer are closely related.

Sensolite® is a therapeutic medical device officially registered in the European Union. It is harmless and without side effects.[26]

PDT

One of the pathways used for cancer treatment today is the use of Photodynamic Therapy (PDT), that is less invasive compared to other methods such as surgery. It makes use of a drug-based agent within a cream. The earliest recorded treatments that exploited a photosensitizer (light sensitive) and a light source (in this case, sunlight) for medical effect can be found in ancient Egyptian and Indian sources.

The first detailed scientific evidence that agents – photosensitive synthetic dyes – in combination with a light source and oxygen could have potential therapeutic effect was made in 1903 in the laboratory of professor H von Tappeiner in Munich, Germany. The observations on the effects of light in 1900 by Oscar Raab, a student of von Tappeiner and the research of Dr A Jesionik were pivotal to the research which showed that oxygen was essential for the 'photodynamic action' – a term coined by von Tappeiner.

Even though von Tappeiner and colleagues went on to perform the first PDT trial in patients with skin carcinoma using the photosensitizer with positive results, it not until the 1970s at the Roswell Park Cancer Institute in the USA that systematic clinical studies on PDT led by Dr Thomas Dougherty were conducted. In 1975 Dougherty *et al* reported that hematoporphyrin derivative (HpD) in combination with red light could completely eradicate mammary tumor growth in rats and mice. The Russian scientists advanced its use clinically, and collaborated with NASA medical scientists from 1992-1998 who were looking at the use of LEDs as more suitable light sources, compared to lasers for PDT applications.

An important factor in the successful use of PDT is that light is needed to activate photosensitizers. Other light-based and laser therapies such as laser wound healing and rejuvenation do not require a photosensitizer.

Existing international research already shows that PDT can be applied in many clinical situations:

- dental: periodontal disease, leukoplakia, gingivitis
- eye: diabetic retinopathy, choroidal neovascularization.
- cardiovascular: anti-angiogenic and anti-atherosclerotic therapies
- lung: respiratory papillomatosis, pseudomonas aeruginosa, mycobacterium tuberculosis, mycobacteriul leprae
- skin: acne, actinic keratoses, basal cell skin carcinoma, candida albicans, cutaneous T cell lymphoma, herpes simplex virus, herpes zoster virus, human papilloma virus, kaposi's scarcoma, leishmaniasis, MRSA, mycobacterium leprae, mycobacterium ulcerans, psoraisis, rosacea, squamous cell carcinoma

PDT is now an established therapy for the treatment of 'wet' neo vascular Age Related Macular Degeneration (AMD) and some other retinal diseases associated with leaky new vessels.

Cancer surgeon Dr Mohammed Keshtgar is applying PDT to selected patients with primary breast cancer at the Royal Free Hospital, London. Keshtgar hopes PDT could be used in place of a lumpectomy and even a mastectomy in certain breast cancer cases.

Successful animal studies using PDT have melted away atherosclerotic plagues, paving the way to significantly reduce the incidence of heart attacks and strokes in humans and may even eliminate the need for coronary bypass surgery in some cases.[27]

PDT has rapidly developed through its first generation and second generation stages.

WHOLE BODY LIGHT CANCER TREATMENT

NGPDT

The newer third generation Next Generation PDT (NGPDT) technology is high-powered light technology that achieves much greater depth of light penetration, therefore allowing deeper penetration and treatment for more invasive cancers. NGPDT is non-toxic and non-invasive and embraces local treatment and systemic whole body treatment.

Some first and second generation PDT agents are derived from synthetic materials that are toxic. This cutting edge development uses a tumor-specific chlorophyll-based photosensitizer to treat a wide variety of solid cancers, including deep tissue and multi-site cancers. This non-toxic plant-based NGPDT agent is designed to utilize high frequency light for deep tumor activation and travel around the body via the blood, only sticking to cancer cells. Due to their greater metabolic activity, tumor cells preferentially take up the photosensitizer compared to normal cells and the NGPDT agent selectively accumulates into cancer cells only, so the light can be safely provided over the whole body, to treat every area affected by the cancer. NGPDT treats most cancers, including:

- anal
- bone
- brain (GBM) and astrocytoma
- breast
- cervical
- colon
- endometrial
- esophagus

- head and neck
- kidney
- liver
- lung
- lymphomas
- pancreas
- penis
- prostate
- skin
- stomach
- tongue
- vaginal

Most modern PDT applications involve 3 key components: a photosensitizer, a light source, and tissue oxygen. The effect of PDT can be localized and specificity of treatment is achieved in 3 ways:

- Light is delivered only to tissues to be treated. In the absence of light, there is no activation of the photosensitizer and no cell killing.
- Photosensitizers may be administered in ways to restrict their mobility.
- Photosensitizers may be chosen which are selectively absorbed at a greater rate by targeted cells.

The fundamental success of NGPDT lies in the ability to penetrate through tissue and bone, up to 20 centimetres, and to selectively attach to malignant tissue and cause singlet oxygen (that is harmful to cancer cells) to be released inside the cancer cell, resulting in either necrosis (immediate cell death) or apoptosis (cells are damaged and will die later), while leaving healthy tissue unaffected. The chemical destruction of tumor cells and vasculature by singlet oxygen is quick.

Post-operative recovery after PDT is typically hours or days rather than weeks. Earlier PDT agents traveled through the body for two or three months. As NGPDT has a 24-hour clearance time in the body, there is no need to keep people in the dark as photosensitivity is not a problem. There is no damage to the immune system.

NGPDT is effective in treating metastatic cancer because even metastatic, microscopic cancer cells that are too small to be seen with traditional diagnostic imaging techniques (PET, CT scan, X-ray) are killed with the whole body treatment with NGPDT.

Treatment

A NGPDT photosynthesizing agent that is sensitive to light is ingested which selectively accumulates and concentrates in malignant cancer tissue. The patient is then exposed to specific light wavelengths in the specialized whole body light delivery system. The specific light activates the agent on the cancer cells causing singlet oxygen to be created, which damages and destroys malignant cancer tissue. Soon after light treatment, the immune system recognizes the fragments of the cancer cells and produces antibodies that help to control and destroy cancer cells throughout the body.

The NGPDT technology utilizes tens of thousands of LEDs. LEDs are advantageous for the treatment of the whole body, as different wavelengths (red and infrared) can be blended in a panel so multiple peaks of absorption for an agent can be activated with one treatment session. Many forms of light are used – LED and deep penetrating laser light. The highest frequency light cannot be seen by the naked eye and the low frequency light is red. NGPDT peak of absorption is in the upper range of 635 nm and higher, which allows light to activate through body tissue and bone, allowing deep tumor treatment therapy.

A stage 1, 2 or 3 cancer typically requires one or two courses of treatment. A stage 4 cancer typically requires two or four courses. As every patient is different, the protocol is duly mediated to suit individual requirements. Recent PET/CT scans and blood tests are required to assess suitability to this treatment. A typical treatment course is:

DAY 1   The patient is reviewed as to suitability and informed of any contraindications prior to any therapy application.

DAY 2   The patient is administered 1mg/kg bodyweight of photosensitive agent.

DAY 3   The patient is administered light via approved light delivery devices.

DAY 4   Following review, the patient is administered a re-supply of the photosensitive agent.

DAY 5   Patient is given light treatments similar to day 3.

DAY 6   Patient is administered agent (re-supply).

DAY 7   Patient is administered light as in day 3 above.

Following the treatment and with the disintegration of tumor cells, the following side effects may appear:

- feeling of tiredness, appearance of cold symptoms along with inflammation and slight aches and malaise in the area of disintegration of the tumors
- slightly high temperature and night sweat may occur for individual patients
- cough may occur for lung cancer patients after receiving treatment
- for the digestive system cancer patients, there may be some diarrhoea or slight bleeding due to necrotic tumor sloughing off
- swelling and inflammation in the area of tumor breakdown.

The side effects are minimal compared to the often harsh side effects from surgical, radiation and chemotherapy treatments for cancer. Chemotherapy suppresses the immune system and NGPDT activates it. Ideally, a patient should allow a period of at least one month after their last chemotherapy, or until the immune system is strong enough before beginning NGPDT.

NGPDT is not suitable for everyone. If tumors are too close to any main artery, the patient is not suitable for treatment as it makes tumors swell before they go smaller. Therefore, many patients with brain tumors are not suitable for treatment. If the immune system is too low, the treatment is not suitable as it requires an immune response.[28]

PDT technology offers an effective remedy for MRSA and other antibiotic resistant infections because its action is more akin to an antiseptic, directly killing the bacterium. This research used first and second generation technology. NGPDT Global Ltd are researching this area further and developing new therapies for many life-threatening viral infections including HIV, HCV and HPV, as it is well established that PDT is very effective in eliminating a wide variety of pathogens from blood samples. This technology is now also being used for diagnostic purposes for skin, breast and prostate cancers.

NGPDT is approved for use in China, as traditionally the Chinese do not favor toxic therapies. This therapy is currently in use in two hospitals in China and four clinical studies have been published. Trials commenced in Australia in 2012, with the results documented by some of Australia's most senior, internationally recognized cancer experts with the peer review process being performed as per TGA guidelines. Trials are also approved for Vietnam for three common female cancers. NGPDT are also using an interstitial treatment for many late stage cancers via a new guided laser delivery option.

COLORS, CRYSTALS, CHAKRAS

Ancient civilizations held that the healing power of light is found in its component parts, that is, color. Color is our perception of light of different wavelengths. Findings by Dr Smith-Sonneborn have clearly shown that certain types of light are not only capable of assisting cells in repairing their DNA, but also have the ability to stimulate life-extending capabilities within the DNA.[29]

Dr Liberman recounts in *Light: Medicine of the Future*, the emotional lives of patients that have been transformed by working with colors. Liberman looked to the basic tenet of homeopathy, which states that the most appropriate remedy for a patient is one with a vibration that is equivalent to the patient's pathology. He also considered Rife's work, where Rife determined the exact 'color' associated with a particular virus or other infectious agent organism and found that irradiating the organism with the same color of light it gave off would very quickly destroy it.

Liberman noticed that the behavior of patients with addictive personalities became more addictive or less addictive depending on the colors at which they looked. Liberman states when situations in life trigger fear or discomfort, our inability to be present with these feelings, as well as to deal with them, forces us to protect ourselves by avoiding or numbing out the situations and going into an addictive behavior pattern. He states such a behavior pattern may be totally unconscious and believes it to be the basis of all addiction. He noticed that once patients had resolved the emotionally painful issues triggered by the colors, then looking at these colors – which was originally uncomfortable – actually stimulated feelings of joy and euphoria.

Liberman also discovered that the colors to which people were unreceptive correlated almost 100 percent of the time with the portions of their bodies where they housed stress, developed disease, or had injured themselves. He found a person might be uncomfortable looking at the color blue, and during the case history he would discover that this person had chronic sore throats, significant dental problems, difficulty with verbal expression (a function of the throat and mouth) and had his or her tonsils removed.[30] This correlates with ancient Sanskrit writings that synthesize energy centres (chakras) with color. These energy centers are believed to be awakened, balanced and healed by specific vibratory energies whose visible equivalents are colors.

Colors are vibrations that resonate at specific frequencies. Words are a vibrational complex of sound. Thoughts are vibrational and different thoughts vibrate at different frequencies. All aspects of thought – emotion, reason, will and desire – are accompanied by vibrations, which is at the heart of the body-mind connection currently penetrating modern day thinking.

Neurobiologist Dr Candace Pert discovered and proved that 'neuropeptides', which are the chemicals triggered by emotions, are thoughts converted into matter. Pert states the mind and body cannot be seen as separate anymore as it is now proven that the same kinds of cells that manufacture and receive emotional chemistry in the brain are present throughout the body.[31] This correlates with the ancient Hermetic Principle of Mentalism – All is Mind – from the Emerald Tablet.

The recognized influence of light on our behavior and emotional states is bringing forth technology that will change how we resolve health issues and how we live. Psychiatrist Dr Richard Frenkel, who has been investigating and clinically using color to treat human stress since the 1960s, hypothesizes that stress is encoded in the mind as color. Since everything in life is colored, he believes that all our experiences, as well as our reactions to them, are fused into what he calls an Experience Complex and then coded in the mind as specific colors. To Frenkel, the mind acts as a computerized color information bank that stores experiences, both stressful and nonstressful, in their respective colors.[32]

SchoolVision lighting allows teachers to control the classroom atmosphere to create exactly the right ambience and mood. In May 2009, the results of a year-long scientific study by Universitätsklinikum Hamburg-Eppendorf with 166 pupils and 18 teachers showed, by using SchoolVision: reading speed increased by almost 35%, frequency of errors reduced by almost 45%, and hyperactive behavior also dropped by an astonishing 76%.[33]

The Irlen Method is a research-based process that uses colored overlays and filters to improve reading fluency, comprehension, attention and concentration, to help those suffering reading and learning problems, dyslexia, ADD/ADHD, autism, headaches, migraines.[34] Color-coded keyboards for computers minimize movements of hands, wrists and arms which could reduce the incidence of Carpal Tunnel Syndrome and Repetitive Stress Injuries (RSI).[35]

Dr Gabriel Cousens, author of *Spiritual Nutrition* and *The Rainbow Diet*, believes nature has color coded all foods so that we can intuitively and logically understand their specific purposes within our bodies. Using a technique called Vascular Autonomic Signal (VAS), Cousens discovered that different foods nourish different aspects of our being. He noticed that a food's color was directly related to the corresponding energy centre of the same color and that the purpose of a particular food was to energize, balance and heal the corresponding energy center, as well as the glands, organs and nerve centers associated with it. Each food, depending on it its color, has a specific affinity for a particular energy center within the body.

Cousens suggests, since the progression of color in nature throughout the days moves from the red, orange, and yellow of the sunrise to the blue, indigo, and violet of the sunset, to follow this in our eating of colorful foods: red, orange and yellow foods in the morning, yellow, green and blue foods at midday, and blue, indigo, violet and golden foods in the evening.[36]

The doctrine of signatures encourages us to look to the signatures in our foods to assist us in making food choices for our health. How the fruit or vegetable is shaped or colored gives us the keys to what part of the body it will assist: i.e., sliced carrot looks like the human eye, a tomato is red and has four chambers just like the human heart, figs (that are full of seeds and hang in two's on the tree) are believed to increase the motility and numbers of male sperm and to overcome male sterility. Also, as the avocado is shaped like a womb and it takes nine months to grow from blossom to ripened fruit, it is food for the womb.

Liberman explains most foods are light in solid form and the closer our food is to being manufactured directly from light, the closer we are to receiving light's full force: organically grown fruits and vegetables are an example of light-filled foods. Processed foods significantly reduce and/or totally eliminate light's nutritional value within that food. Elixirs and essences will become better understood as we further appreciate Nature's bounty of foods, herbs, flowers and gems.

Dr Hazel Parcells feels that color is the body's life-force: color can change any function of the body. In cases of illness or exhaustion, she finds that the flow of color to the body's organs is reduced until health is restored. Neonatal jaundice is believed by some researchers to be caused by immaturity of the infant's organs, although lack of sunlight may be an important factor. Babies with jaundice have been treated with blue light (450nm) since the 1960s. Blue light is also used for rheumatoid arthritis. During the birth process, Parcells applies color treatments to both mother and infant to reduce shock, hemorrhage and recovery time. She finds that color can, in many stroke cases, successfully eliminate paralysis and fully restore normal function.

Dr Barbara Parry has shown women treated with two hours of bright light in the evening have experienced a reversal of their premenstrual syndrome (PMS) symptoms. For men, the recent development of the GreenLight PVP laser prostatectomy system, using the LBO crystal instead of the KTP crystal, has had significant implications for urologists and their patients, as it literally vaporizes tissue and simultaneously seals the tissue, resulting in an almost bloodless field for Benign Prostatic Hyperplasia (BPH).

Crystals

Writings on the Atlantean civilization propose crystals were used in all facets of living, well beyond our present-day achievements. Our growing knowledge on the use of crystals to transmute and transform electromagnetic energy has revolutionized our way of living with the evolution of newer technologies. Silicon, an artificially grown crystal, is used to create solar cells, enabling us to harness the energies of sunlight to power these technologies. Silicon solar cells are also found in calculators and watches. A ruby crystal was a key component in the first laser developed by Bell Laboratory scientists in the early 1960s. Ordinarily, light is incoherent, with rays of energy moving randomly in many directions at once. In the ruby laser, the crystal creates an amplification effect by organizing rays of light into a coherent, orderly beam that has a tremendously powerful energetic effect. The quartz crystal works similarly with the subtle energies of the healer.[37]

Quartz crystals are used in many electronic devices today and in communications and information storage. They are also used for healing. As a rule, the healing energies transmitted by crystals seem to work at the level of our subtle energetic bodies.[38]

Gerber suggests in order to therapeutically alter our subtle bodies, we must administer energy that vibrates at frequencies beyond the physical plane. Gerber further states, quartz crystals are thought-energy amplifiers and operate at the level beyond the speed of light (negative space/time).[39] The Jivaro in South America and the tribes of Australia consider the quartz crystal the strongest power object of all.[40]

Science has recently begun to explore the 'liquid crystal' and, as our understanding of artificially created liquid crystals has grown, so have biologists come to recognize that many of the cellular membranes and structures within the human body are liquid crystal as well. A number of solid and liquid crystalline structures at the physical level are involved in the attunement of subtle energies within the nervous system and the flow of the life-force through the body.[41]

Oschman states all therapeutic and scientific approaches to the body can benefit from an appreciation of the crystalline nature of living tissues: crystalline arrangements are the rule and not the exception in living systems. Healers who use crystalline materials (quartz, shells, stones) believe they enhance the effectiveness of their work. Oschman explains crystalline objects have resonant interactions with the highly ordered liquid crystals within the tissues of the therapist and the person being touched. In other words, crystals enhance vibratory energy exchanges between two individuals.[42]

In the words of Dr William Tiller PhD, one of the leading theorists in the subtle energetic field:

Just as metals are keys to electricity, so crystals are keys to this new development of the use of energy. The magnet is the Matter polarity and crystals are the Spirit polarity. Creativity takes place always between two polarities. Therefore, the right combination of magnets and crystals will produce the creative effect of energy. Light on the crystal and magnet, that is, lines of force from the magnet are the components of a new energy system.[43]

Tiller states the atomic bomb is a destructive way to unlocking energy – the left-hand path method – and crystals are the right-hand path method.

Chakras

The endocrine glands are part of a powerful master control system, affecting the physiology of the body from the level of cellular gene activation up to the functioning of the central nervous system. Ancient Sanskrit writings describe the body as having a series of seven major energy centers known as chakras (wheels of light), which are located approximately at the sites of the major endocrine glands in the physical body:

ENERGY CENTER	CHAKRA	GLAND	COLOR
Crown	Crown	Pineal	Violet
Brow	Ajna	Pituitary	Indigo
Throat	Vishuddha	Thyroid, Parathyroid	Blue
Heart	Anahata	Thymus	Green
Solar Plexus	Manipura	Adrenals, Pancreas	Yellow
Sacral	Svadisthana	Splenic	Orange
Root	Muladhara	Gonads	Red

EPILOGUE

LIGHT YEARS AHEAD

Trying to understand the absolute laws of the cosmos by the process of intellectualizing, the ancients observed the individual, collective cycles, and rhythms of the celestial bodies. The virgin Moon in the darkness with its cycles enables the birth of the Sun against the backdrop of the blue cloak of the sky. The Moon, the stars, and the Sun, somehow all danced together as One in a harmonious recurring cycle.

These events gave rise to story upon story, which layered upon layers to the countless myths and religions that abound in our world today. In order to make simple the great truths of Nature and the abstract principles of Natural Law, the vital forces of the universe were personified, becoming the gods and goddesses of the ancient mythologies.[1] The ancients, like all of us, were looking for an answer to the riddle of life and the Source of All.

It is the spark, in the form of light that ignites the process of living. Ott states the human body requires fuel (in the form of food), oxygen, and a spark (in the form of light) to ignite the process of metabolism and there is no question in his mind that the visible portion of the spectrum, as well as certain portions beyond, especially the ultraviolet, act as the ignition system for all human biological functions.[2]

All ancient philosophies and open medical systems acknowledge an all-pervading life force which runs timelessly through life. Continuously active within us, this subtle energy is termed: *'nous'* (Egyptian), *'chi'* (Chinese), *'ki'* (Japanese), *'prana'* (Indian), and *'chitta'* (Vedic). In 1925, Georges Lakhovsky stated that human DNA vibrated or resonated at 50+GHz. In 1982, Ukrainian nuclear physicists began studying the effects of application of human DNA frequencies to specific acupuncture points. They determined that human DNA resonates at 54-78 GHz. Quantum physicists report that the Sun bathes the Earth with 52-78 GHz energy, among others. Thus, solar energy is a major factor in maintaining life energy (*chi*) – DNA resonance.[3]

There also exists however another energy, the underlying energy of creation, which has existed since the beginning. Following on from the famous mathematician and astronomer and one of the greatest scientists of all time, Pierre-Simon Laplace (1749–1827), physicist James Clerk Maxwell (1831–1879) furthered the concept of scalar waves, laying the foundation for quantum physics. This 'energy' was accidentally discovered by Nikola Tesla (1856–1943) who termed it 'radiant energy'. The term 'scalar wave' which originates from mathematics is also referred to as a Tesla wave.

Tesla warned of the dangers of X-ray radiation and learned how to harness scalar energy from one transmitter to another without using any wires. Tesla planned to utilize scalar energy as the preferred carrier wave for all telecommunications. There has been resistance accepting the existence of scalar waves as many scientists and individuals only think of the measurable as real: what they cannot measure, cannot exist.

Albert Einstein (1879–1955), considered the most influential physicist of the 20th century, documented how scalar waves could be practically applied. Scalar energy is now also referred to as a 'torsion field' and zero point energy.

Today, scalar technology is utilized for communication systems and also used in locating humans and other animals during rescue-search operations. A scalar energy instrument was also used to track and monitor the Apollo 11 astronauts during their lunar mission by way of their photographs. With Tesla's discovery and the recent discoveries of Professor Konstantin Meyl, considered by many to be a modern-day Tesla, the utilization of scalar waves can bring forth a reality of wireless transportation of electric energy and communications.[4] Imagine a world without pollution, as cars will be charged through the air as they drive. A world where there is no electrosmog and no harmful effects on life on Earth.

Oschman comments scalar energy appears to: interact with atomic nuclei rather than with electrons and be intimately involved in healing.[5] In contrast to the electromagnetic wave, a scalar wave transports energy in addition to the information. Scalar is non-linear, exists in a dimension where there is no time or space and does not decay with time or distance. Cells and tissues are highly non-linear, cooperative, and coherent systems.[6]

It is written that Antoine Priore (1912–1983) utilized a powerful and accurate scalar energy instrument that effectively reprogrammed the mutated DNA in both humans and animals alike, and subsequently cured all types of cancer. Thomas Galen Hieronymus (1895-1988) observed that each organ or tissue in the human body possessed a unique scalar energy harmonic and that the level of vitality of an organ or tissue could likewise be ascertained by way of scalar energy analysis.[7]

EPILOGUE — LIGHT YEARS AHEAD

The 20th century witnessed the 'cracking' of the human DNA code. Spurred on by the work of scientist Rosalind Franklin, American biologist James Watson and English biochemist Francis Crick discovered DNA's double-helix structure in 1953. Today we know, just as certain aspects of the human energy system have the same transformational properties as natural quartz crystals, our DNA shares characteristics with scalar energy.

Meyl recently detected that our whole body works with scalar waves and furthers that the brain is a scalar wave computer, information that will take us light years ahead, reflecting the Theogenic Idea: 'taking off where the gods left off'. In theory, practising alchemy: taking something that already exists and improving on it – imitating Nature and surpassing it.[8]

Effectively enhancing the scalar environment within and around us has the ability to override the artificial EMF we have created and assist in our physical and emotional well-being. This predominant energy of the universe, that gives us the brilliant yellow hues of sunflowers to the burnt scarlet shades of sunsets, is often referred to as 'divine light'.

APPENDIX

APPENDIX A

LEGAL ADVICE
TO THE POWER INDUSTRY

WATSON & RENNER Privileged Attorney-Client Communication

14 June 2007
FOR: UHSG Members
RE: EMF Science Reviews

We attach an updated list of EMF science reviews conducted by scientific panels, public health organizations, or governmental bodies. Since 1977, there have been 113 such reviews. The attached report lists these reviews, along with representative conclusions from each review. While each review includes many conclusions, the quotes from each review are representative of the overall conclusions(s) reached in that review.

We believe this list of science reviews and their key conclusions is useful information to consider in assessing the development of the EMF issue, and in preparing public disclosures and communications materials.

In the past, it was possible to preface the list with a statement that:

> "none of these reviews has concluded that exposure to power-frequency EMF causes cancer or any other disease."

We believe such a representation is no longer advisable because of the release of the California Department of Health (CDHS) "Fourth and Final Draft" report on EMF research (see #111 on attached list). The CDHS draft report concludes in part that:

> "To one degree or another all three of the DHS scientists are inclined to believe that EMFs <u>can cause</u> some degree of increased risk of childhood leukemia, adult brain cancer, Lou Gehrig's Disease, and miscarriage." (Emphasis added).

The final CDHS report is expected to contain the same statement.

It is possible to argue that the CDHS conclusion does not say explicitly that there is an established cause and effect relationship between EMF and any disease. We believe, however that the CDHS conclusion is sufficiently close to causation that a global statement that none of the science reviews concludes there is a causal relationship would be legally inadvisable.

1919 M Street, NW, Washington, DC 20036 Tel: 202 737 6302
Crenner@W-R.com Fax: 202 737 7611

APPENDIX B

SANITARY NORMS MANDATE
THE REPUBLIC OF KAZAKHSTAN

CONFIRMED:
The order of the Head State Sanitary Physician of the Republic of Kazakhstan
28 November 2003 r.No.69

Permissible levels of high-frequency electromagnetic pollutions' voltage in a wires of industrial frequency alternating current

Sanitary-epidemiologic norms

1 – General provisions

1. Sanitary-and-epidemiologic norms «Permissible levels of high-frequency electromagnetic pollutions' voltage in a wires of industrial frequency alternating current" (further – norms) define levels electromagnetic pollutions in electric wires of power supply of an industrial electric equipment, office techniques, electrical household appliances in a range 1 kiloHertz – 400 kiloHertz (further – kHz).

2. The present norms are directed on improvement and optimization of a sanitary-epidemiologic situation and prevention of environmental contamination by electromagnetic radiation, and also management of corresponding risk, in addition to existing norms.

3. Heads of the organizations and physical persons which activity is connected to operation of the industrial organizations using the equipment and devices, being sources of electromagnetic radiation, provide maintenance of requirements of the present norms.

4. In the present norms the following terms and definitions are used: electromagnetic pollution – parasitic (casual) frequencies in a network of an alternating current of industrial frequency of 50 Hertz (further – Hz) which source is not determined; electromagnetic pollutions – one of kinds of electromagnetic pollution in a range of frequencies 1 kHz–400 kHz, arising in networks of an alternating current of industrial frequency.

2 – Permissible level of electromagnetic pollutions' voltage

5. The permissible level of a high-frequency electromagnetic pollutions' voltage in a range of frequencies 1 kHz–400 kHz in a wires of an alternating current of industrial frequency of 50 Hz should not exceed 0,05 volts (further – V) 50 millivolts (further – mV).

3 – Choice of points of the control

6. Control points get out in the socket of wires of an alternating current of industrial frequency (50 Hz), taking place near to a plug (socket) of a cable

of the connected equipment. The number of control points depends on number of workplaces. In each control point one measurement is carried out.

4 – Recommended devices for the control

7. For the control high-frequency electromagnetic pollutions in a range of frequencies (1-400) kHz in a wires of an alternating current of industrial frequency of 50 Hz are recommended to be used millivoltmeter, having corresponding characteristics and registered in the State Register of Republic of Kazakhstan.

5 – Requirements to carrying out of measurement

8. The device is plugged into socket of an alternating current in a control point.

9. Tap switch of ranges necessary to put in position of 1–2 V.

10. If indications are not fixed or are small, tap switch put in position 100–999 mV or in position 1,1-99,9 mV, depending on a registered level of a voltage. Results are registered and compared to the norms specified in item 5 of the present norms.

Note by Donna Fisher:
Point 5. Where it states 50 millivolts this should state 50 GS units. This has occurred as the new term of GS units did not exist in 2003 resulting in a translation inaccuracy.

APPENDIX C

Dirty Electricity

Prior to 1972, most electrical loads were linear – that is, they operated on normal utility supplied 50/60 Hertz sine waves. Linear loads include devices such as motors and incandescent light bulbs. Non-linear loads use short pulses of current. Therefore, load current is not proportional to the voltage applied. When load current and voltage are not proportional entities, harmonics are generated and flow on the power distribution lines.

Dirty electricity is poor power quality and refers to an electrical signal that deviates from a normal 50/60 Hz sine wave. The technical term for dirty electricity – an unwanted modulation that is contaminating our electrical supply – is 'high-frequency voltage transients', as it rides along our electrical wiring. Dirty electricity can be picked up by the power lines delivering electricity to the home from the utility. Incorrect wiring, poor power quality, unbalanced electrical loads and interruptions to the flow of electrical current create continuous spikes (transients) up into this higher and more hazardous frequency.

Dirty electricity can even extend into radio frequencies above several MHz and can often get into the microwave range of the electromagnetic spectrum. Virtually all of today's energy-efficient electronic devices are drawing their needs intermittently, inducing high levels of high-frequency harmonics and distortion back into a building's electrical system thus creating dirty electricity. Devices are using more pulsed power and various forms of switching power supplies with transformers that convert our AC current to the low-voltage DC power used to power all our electronics. The appliances convert the AC they are receiving to DC, which the equipment will use to power its activities using less electricity. In this process, high frequencies are produced that go out onto the electrical circuit and cause high-frequency electromagnetic waves to radiate out from the circuits.

Some of the high frequencies produced are radiowave and microwave frequencies that disseminate their energy through the air rather than follow the electrical circuits. Dirty electricity is also the result of interrupted current generated by electrical appliances and equipment resulting in spikes. In the process of saving energy, these energy-efficient DC devices chop up the conventional AC 50/60 Hz sine waves and create electrical transients.

Transients are large, very brief increases in voltage: distortions in the sine wave that occur when electrical equipment is switched on and off, interrupting the electrical current flow. Transients have the effect of creating a high-frequency signal that is superimposed on the 50/60 Hz signal, creating 'parasitic oscillations' that ride on top of the existing 50/60 Hz power.

Examples of modern-day equipment designed to operate with interrupted current flow are: dimmer switches, which interrupt the current twice per cycle, or 120 times per second (it takes a lot of electrical energy to dim the light, and this 'excess light' is converted to radio frequencies), energy-efficient compact fluorescent lighting (20,000 times per second), halogen lamps, and all equipment produced since the 1980s that uses switching power supplies.

The more that electricity deviates from the 50/60 Hz sine wave the poorer the power quality and the more dirty the electricity. High-frequency dirty electricity generated by electrical equipment in buildings travels along the electrical distribution system in and between buildings and through the ground. Dirty electricity generated outside the building enters the building on electrical wiring and through ground rods and conductive plumbing. Humans and conducting objects in contact with the ground become part of the circuit.

The STETZERiZER filter contains an electrical capacitor that shorts out the harmful high-frequency transients and harmonics on the circuit that contributes to poor power quality.

Computers generate at higher frequencies and the power surges occurred due to our 50/60 Hz wiring being polluted by these higher frequencies. What is now known is that this energy from the computer is coupled to our bodies by the capacitance – a measure of the capacitor's ability to store charge – between our bodies and the electrical wires within the walls of our buildings. These higher frequencies are more likely to penetrate living organisms as they have more energy than ELF EMF in the 50/60 Hz range. Energy is proportional to frequency: the energy is 1,000 times higher at 60 kHz than it is at 60 Hz. These surges of radio-frequency energy can contain up to 2,500 times the energy of 50/60 Hz.

The STETZERiZER Meter

Specifically, the meter measures the average magnitude of the changing voltage as a function of time (dV/dt), which naturally emphasizes transients and other high frequency phenomena that change rapidly with time. The measurements of dV/dt read by the meter are defined as GS units. The GS units are a measure of 'harmful energy' which is a function of frequency, or more generally, rate of change of voltage or dV/dt. The meter measures the current in an 800 picofarad capacitor connected across the terminals of the outlet into which it is plugged.

One GS unit is 0.02 microamperes. A meter reading of 50 would indicate a current of one microampere. A human having a low impedance to one of the terminals of the outlet (the grounded wire) and a capacitive coupling of 800 picofarads to wiring connected to the other terminal of the outlet (the hot wire) would have a current flowing through them indicated by the meter. The capacitance of two parallel metal plates that are one meter by one meter and separated by one centimetre is about 800 picofarads. The capacitance of a human to the hot wires will usually be less than 800 picofarads and the current through the human will be proportionately lower. The current flow through the human will also depend on how the capacitance of the human to the wire is distributed over the human. This is important since it is the current flowing inside the body and where it is flowing that determines the effect it will have on the human.

The meter is calibrated to the oscilloscope. The Oscilloscope measures the actual waveform usually between two points or potentials. The STETZERiZER meter measures the high frequency energy that is on a building's wires. It also measures this potential between two points. The Positron meter is measuring fields coming through space.

Oscilloscope tracings: Presence and removal of dirty electricity

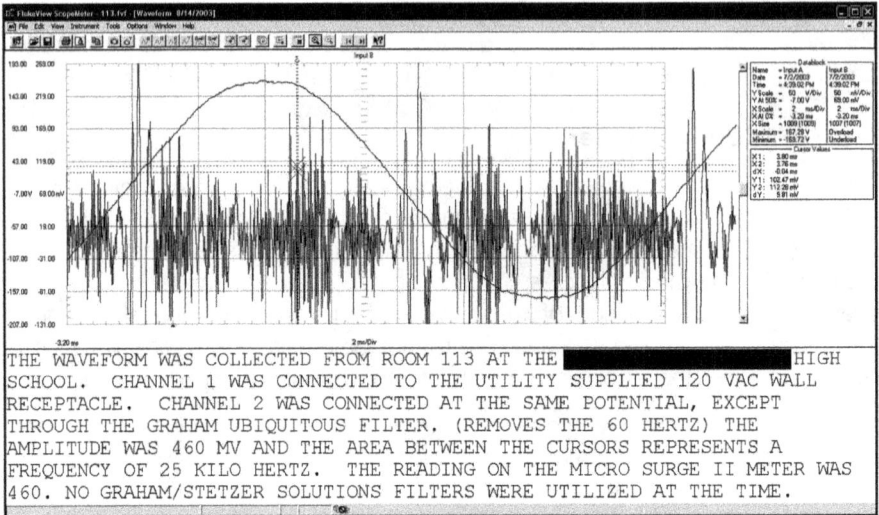

THE WAVEFORM WAS COLLECTED FROM ROOM 113 AT THE ██████████ HIGH
SCHOOL. CHANNEL 1 WAS CONNECTED TO THE UTILITY SUPPLIED 120 VAC WALL
RECEPTACLE. CHANNEL 2 WAS CONNECTED AT THE SAME POTENTIAL, EXCEPT
THROUGH THE GRAHAM UBIQUITOUS FILTER. (REMOVES THE 60 HERTZ) THE
AMPLITUDE WAS 460 MV AND THE AREA BETWEEN THE CURSORS REPRESENTS A
FREQUENCY OF 25 KILO HERTZ. THE READING ON THE MICRO SURGE II METER WAS
460. NO GRAHAM/STETZER SOLUTIONS FILTERS WERE UTILIZED AT THE TIME.

Figure 1: Presence of dirty electricity – 460 GS units

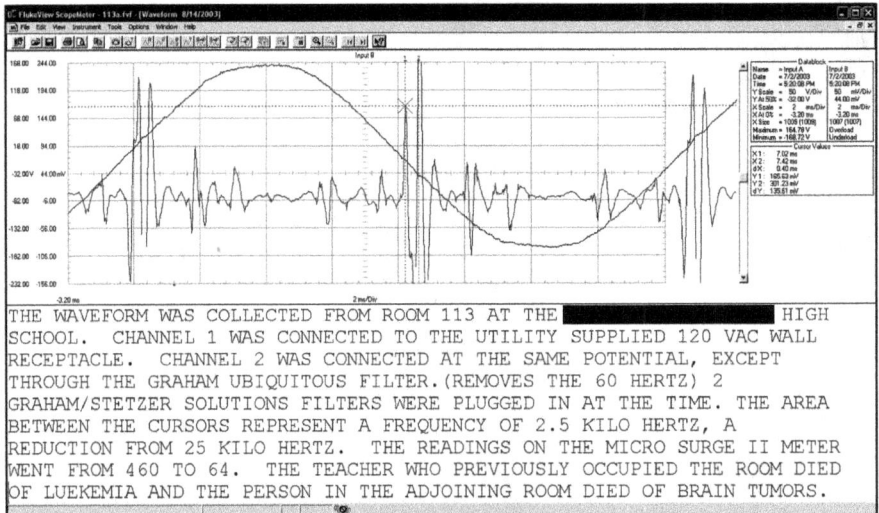

THE WAVEFORM WAS COLLECTED FROM ROOM 113 AT THE ██████████ HIGH
SCHOOL. CHANNEL 1 WAS CONNECTED TO THE UTILITY SUPPLIED 120 VAC WALL
RECEPTACLE. CHANNEL 2 WAS CONNECTED AT THE SAME POTENTIAL, EXCEPT
THROUGH THE GRAHAM UBIQUITOUS FILTER.(REMOVES THE 60 HERTZ) 2
GRAHAM/STETZER SOLUTIONS FILTERS WERE PLUGGED IN AT THE TIME. THE AREA
BETWEEN THE CURSORS REPRESENT A FREQUENCY OF 2.5 KILO HERTZ, A
REDUCTION FROM 25 KILO HERTZ. THE READINGS ON THE MICRO SURGE II METER
WENT FROM 460 TO 64. THE TEACHER WHO PREVIOUSLY OCCUPIED THE ROOM DIED
OF LUEKEMIA AND THE PERSON IN THE ADJOINING ROOM DIED OF BRAIN TUMORS.

Figure 2: Removal of dirty electricity – 64 GS units

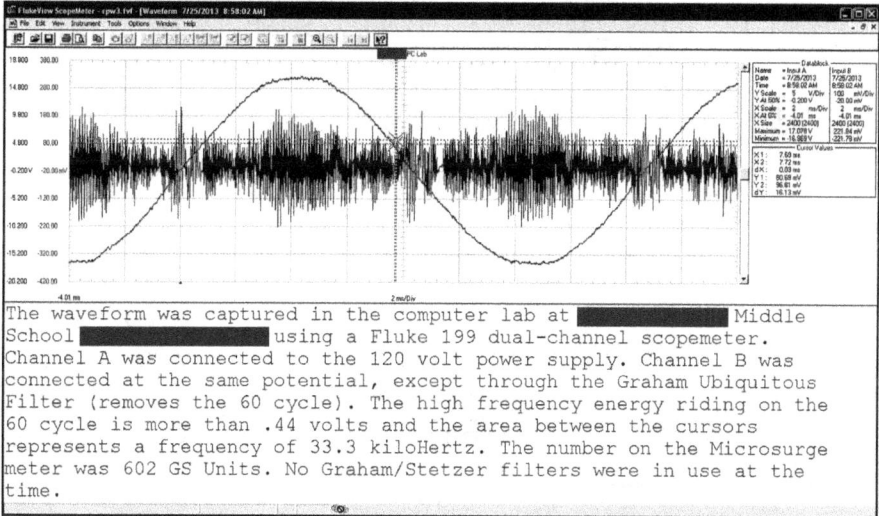

The waveform was captured in the computer lab at ███████████ Middle School ███████████ using a Fluke 199 dual-channel scopemeter. Channel A was connected to the 120 volt power supply. Channel B was connected at the same potential, except through the Graham Ubiquitous Filter (removes the 60 cycle). The high frequency energy riding on the 60 cycle is more than .44 volts and the area between the cursors represents a frequency of 33.3 kiloHertz. The number on the Microsurge meter was 602 GS Units. No Graham/Stetzer filters were in use at the time.

Figure 3: Presence of dirty electricity – 602 GS units

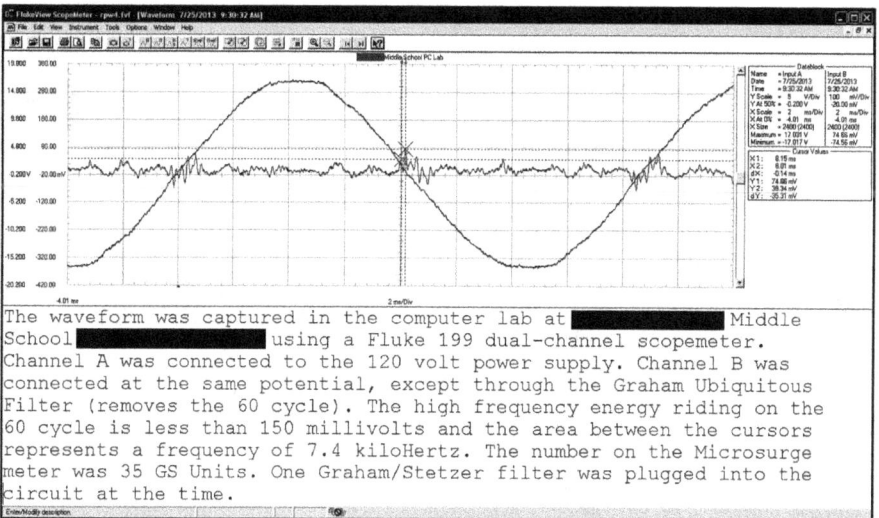

The waveform was captured in the computer lab at ███████████ Middle School ███████████ using a Fluke 199 dual-channel scopemeter. Channel A was connected to the 120 volt power supply. Channel B was connected at the same potential, except through the Graham Ubiquitous Filter (removes the 60 cycle). The high frequency energy riding on the 60 cycle is less than 150 millivolts and the area between the cursors represents a frequency of 7.4 kiloHertz. The number on the Microsurge meter was 35 GS Units. One Graham/Stetzer filter was plugged into the circuit at the time.

Figure 4: Removal of dirty electricity – 35 GS units

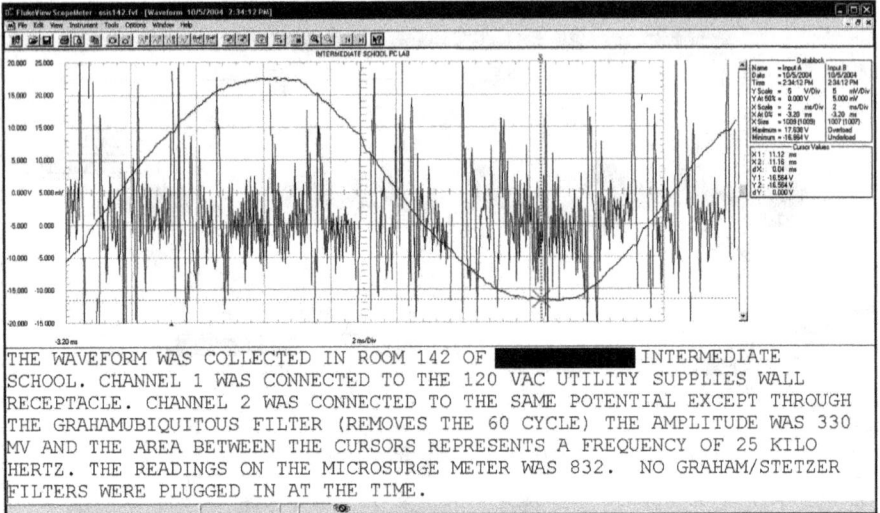

THE WAVEFORM WAS COLLECTED IN ROOM 142 OF ████████████ INTERMEDIATE SCHOOL. CHANNEL 1 WAS CONNECTED TO THE 120 VAC UTILITY SUPPLIES WALL RECEPTACLE. CHANNEL 2 WAS CONNECTED TO THE SAME POTENTIAL EXCEPT THROUGH THE GRAHAMUBIQUITOUS FILTER (REMOVES THE 60 CYCLE) THE AMPLITUDE WAS 330 MV AND THE AREA BETWEEN THE CURSORS REPRESENTS A FREQUENCY OF 25 KILO HERTZ. THE READINGS ON THE MICROSURGE METER WAS 832. NO GRAHAM/STETZER FILTERS WERE PLUGGED IN AT THE TIME.

Figure 5: Presence of dirty electricity – 832 GS units

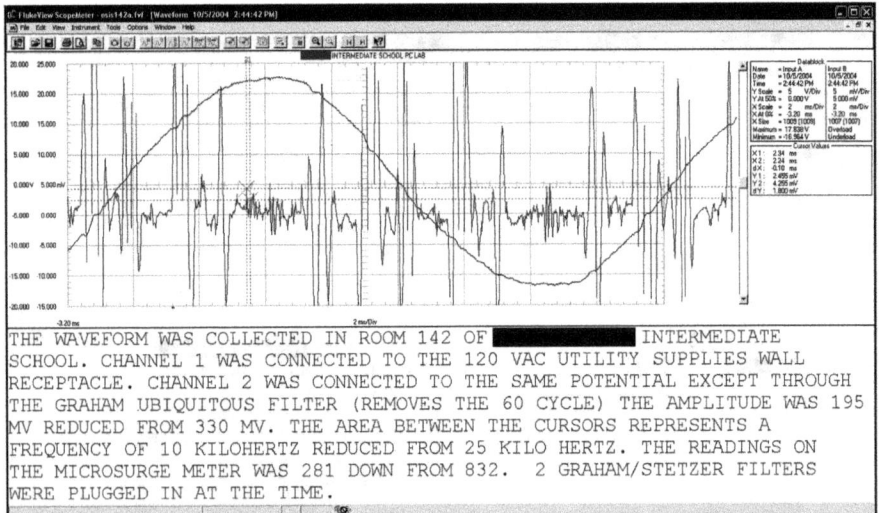

THE WAVEFORM WAS COLLECTED IN ROOM 142 OF ████████████ INTERMEDIATE SCHOOL. CHANNEL 1 WAS CONNECTED TO THE 120 VAC UTILITY SUPPLIES WALL RECEPTACLE. CHANNEL 2 WAS CONNECTED TO THE SAME POTENTIAL EXCEPT THROUGH THE GRAHAM UBIQUITOUS FILTER (REMOVES THE 60 CYCLE) THE AMPLITUDE WAS 195 MV REDUCED FROM 330 MV. THE AREA BETWEEN THE CURSORS REPRESENTS A FREQUENCY OF 10 KILOHERTZ REDUCED FROM 25 KILO HERTZ. THE READINGS ON THE MICROSURGE METER WAS 281 DOWN FROM 832. 2 GRAHAM/STETZER FILTERS WERE PLUGGED IN AT THE TIME.

Figure 6: Removal of dirty electricity – 281 GS units

APPENDIX D : ELECTROMAGNETIC SPECTRUM

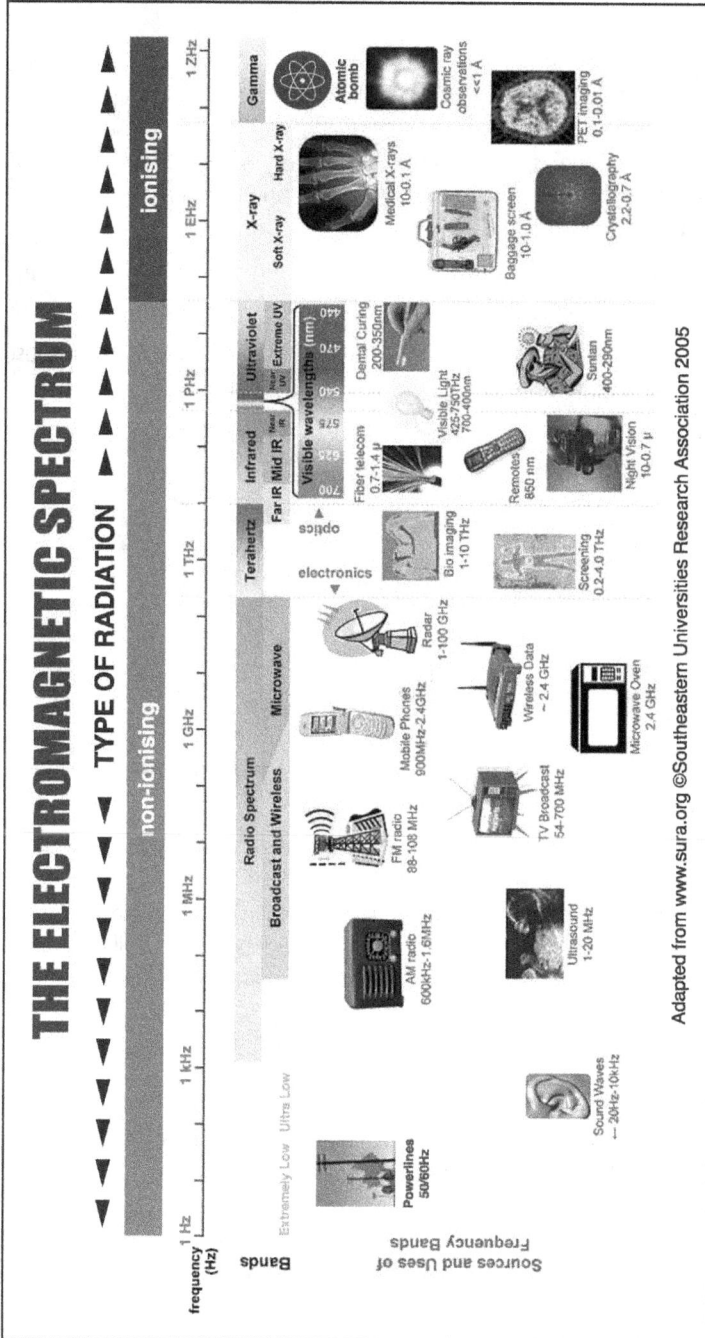

Adapted from www.sura.org ©Southeastern Universities Research Association 2005

GLOSSARY

alchemy: At the physical level, the transmutation of lead into gold. On a spiritual level, this process represents the transformation of the physical personality into an expression of the Higher Self.

blood-brain barrier (BBB): Composition of the fluid that surrounds and protects the brain. The breach of the blood-brain barrier is very dangerous.

cancer cluster: A greater than expected number of cases of a particular disease in a group of people in a geographical area, or over a period of time.

capacitive coupling: Use of a capacitor to transfer energy from one circuit to another.

carcinogenic: Cancer causing – capable of causing cancer.

contact current: Current passed into a biological medium via a contacting electrode or other source of current.

DECTs: Digitally enhanced cordless phones.

dirty power: Term used by the power industry The alternate term used by the scientists is dirty electricity.

electrical pollution: Contributors to Electrical Pollution include: harmonics, transients, sags, swells.

electrohypersensitivity (EHS): A condition where individuals experience adverse health effects while using or being in the vicinity of devices emanating electric, magnetic or electromagnetic fields (EMF). Whatever its cause, EHS is a real and sometimes debilitating problem for the affected persons, while the level of EMF in their neighbourhood is no greater than is encountered in normal living environments.

electromagnetic spectrum: A group of distinct energy forms that emanate from various sources: the energies released are referred to as types of EMR.

ELF: Extremely low frequency (often termed extra-low frequency). The newer term, weak low intensity EMF, is also being used.

ELF EMF: Covers the frequency range of 3–300Hz.

EMF: Electric, magnetic and electromagnetic fields associated with electricity, whether it is from artificially created (man-made) sources such as power generation or from natural processes going on within animal or plant cells.

EME: Electromagnetic energy (often used for EMF/EMR).

energy medicine: The application of physics in the diagnosis & treatment of illness.

epidemiology: A study of the various factors influencing the occurrence, distribution, prevention and control of disease, injury, and other health-related events in a defined human population. Epidemiological studies imply the analysis of a statistical connection between exposure and disease. A statistical connection does not mean that the exposure causes the disease.

femtocell: A femtocell is a small cellular base station designed for use in residential or small business environments. It connects to the service provider's network via a broadband (such as DSL or cable) and typically supports 2 to 5 mobile phones in a residential setting.

free radical: Any atom or molecule with a single unpaired electron in its outer shell.

frequency: The number of complete cycles of an electromagnetic wave in a second. Unit: hertz. Abbreviation: Hz. 1 Hz = 1 cycle per second.

genotoxic: Any evidence of genetic damage, cell death or neoplastic transformation. Any substance that damages DNA or chromosomes. A genotoxic substance is mutagenic, carcinogenic and teratogenic. Genotoxic substances can cause cancer, reproductive health effects and neurological damage.

glioma tumor: Glioblastoma is a very aggressive and fatal brain tumor.

harmonic: Multiples of the original frequency.

ionizing radiation: Electromagnetic radiation with photon energy, high enough to break molecular bonds and damage genetic material. e.g. Gamma rays, X-rays.

liquid crystal: Have a structure which is partially crystalline and partially fluid.

malillumination: Coined by Dr John Ott, it describes the current 'sunlight deprivation and vitamin D starvation' epidemic.

milliGauss; mGauss; mG: Measurement of a magnetic field. A milliGauss is a measure of ELF intensity, and is used to describe electromagnetic fields from appliances, power lines, interior electrical wiring, etc.

milliSievert (mSv); Sievert: attempts to reflect the biological effects of radiation as opposed to the physical aspects. One mSv is equal to one thousandth of a sievert.

mitogen: A chemical substance that encourages a cell to commence cell division, triggering mitosis.

morphic resonance: Memory is inherent in nature

mutagenic: Capable of inducing mutation or increasing its rate.

MW; microwave: Technology that operates at this frequency includes: mobile phones, microwaves, telecommunications links, radar, satellite communications, weather-observation equipment and medical diathermy. Because microwaves are also used for communication, RF and MW emissions overlap considerably. Microwave energy is within the radio frequency band of the electromagnetic spectrum and ranges from 300 MHz–300 GHz.

nanometer: Unit of measurement for the wavelength of electromagnetic radiation and is equivalent to one billionth of a meter.

non-ionizing radiation: The part of the electromagnetic spectrum extending from zero frequency to the frequencies of visible light.

phototherapy: Consists of exposure to daylight or to specific wavelengths of light using polychromatic polarized light, lasers, LEDS, fluorescent lamps, dichroic lamps or very bright, full-spectrum light, usually controlled with various devices. The light is administered for a prescribed amount of time. Classically referred to as heliotherapy.

piezoelectric effect: The ability of certain materials to generate an electric charge in response to applied mechanical stress. Is the property of quartz that we utilize in our receiver and transmitter crystals.

precautionary principle: The principle states that when there are indications of possible adverse effects, though they remain uncertain, the risks from doing nothing may be far greater than the risks of taking action to control these exposures. The precautionary principle shifts the burden of proof from those suspecting a risk to those who discount it.

radar: Radar system has a transmitter that emits either microwaves or radiowaves that are reflected by the target and detected by a receiver.

radiation absorbed dose (RAD): A measurement that calculates the amount of radiation absorbed by body tissues.

radiation: The energy transmitted by waves that travels and spreads out as it goes.

radio frequency radiation (RFR): Generally recognized in the range of approximately 3 kHz–300 GHz.

resonance: The tuning of a biological response to an external signal. Resonance can also be applicable to organs, tissues or other body parts.

rouleaux: Rouleaux formation is when red blood cells stack on to each other due to an abnormal shape, yielding an appearance similar to a stack of coins.

Schumann resonances: Principal background (harmonic) in the electromagnetic spectrum being 7.83 Hz (fundamental), and approximately 14 Hz, 20 Hz, 26 Hz, 33 Hz, 39 Hz, 45 Hz.

specific absorption rate (SAR): Measures the time rate of absorption of electromagnetic energy by the body.

strand break: When a DNA chain breaks apart. **single-strand break:** When the break is in one strand of the DNA's double helix. **double-strand break:** A break occurs on both strands of the DNA's double helix.

teratogenic: Of, relating to, or causing malformations or defects to an embryo or fetus.

transient: A transient is a sub-cycle disturbance in the AC waveform that is evidenced by a sharp but brief discontinuity in the waveform. May be of either polarity and may be additive to or subtractive from the nominal waveform.

µW/cm2: Radio frequency radiation in terms of power density is measured in microwatts per centimeter squared and abbreviated (µW/cm2). It is used when talking about emissions from wireless facilities and when describing ambient RF in the environment.

waveform: The variation of an electrical amplitude with time.

BIBLIOGRAPHY

PUBLICATIONS

Becker RO, Cross Currents: *A Startling Look at the Effects of Electromagnetic Radiation on Your Health: The Perils of Electropollution, the Promise of Electromedicine,* Tarcher Putnam, USA 1990.

Bellamy I, MacLean D, *Radiant Healing: The Many Paths to Personal Harmony and Planetary Wholeness,* Joshua Books, AUS 2005.

BioInitiative Working Group, Cindy Sage and David O Carpenter, Editors, *BioInitiative Report: A Rationale for Biologically-based Public Exposure Standards for Electromagnetic Radiation* at www.bioinitiative.org, 2007.

Blank M, PhD, *Overpowered: What Science Tells Us About the Dangers of Cell Phones and Other WiFi-Age Devices, Seven Stories Press,* USA, 2014.

Bohm D, *Of Matter and Meaning: The Super-Implicate Order, ReVision,* Spring 1983.

Bohm D, *Of Matter and Meaning: The Super-Implicate Order, ReVision,* Spring 1983.

Chandler WB, *Ancient Future: The Teachings and Prophetic Wisdom of the Seven Hermetic Laws of Ancient Egypt,* Black Classic Press, USA 1999.

Coghill R, *The Healing Energies of Light,* Gaia Books, UK 2000.

Davies J, *There are risks as well as benefits – so get the facts, then decide, The Scotsman,* Scotland 2009.

Elwardt HA, *Let's Stop the #1 Killer of Americans Today A Natural Approach to Preventing & Reversing Heart Disease,* Lightning Source Inc, USA 2006.

Eisenstein M with Miller NZ, *Make an Informed Vaccine Decision For the Health of Your Child: A Parent's Guide to Childhood Shots,* New Atlantean Press, Sante Fe, New Mexico, USA 2010.

Epstein SD, Bertell R, Seaman B, *Dangers and Unreliability of Mammography: Breast examination is a safe, effective, and practical alternative,* International Journal of Health Services 31(3): 605-615, 2001.

Evans N, (ed) State of the Evidence: *What is the connection between the environment and breast cancer?,* The Breast Cancer Fund, USA 2004.

Firstenberg A, *The Largest Biological Experiment Ever, Sun Monthly,* January 2006.

Florendo JG Dr, *A Practical Guide To The Benefits Of Scalar Energy,* for The Open Heart Foundation 2010.

Genuis SJ, *Fielding a current idea: Exploring the public health impact of electromagnetic radiation*, Public Health (2007), doi:10.1016/j.puhe. 007.04.008.

Gerber R, MD, *Vibrational Medicine: The #1 Handbook of Subtle-Energy Therapies*, Third Edition, Bear & Company, USA 2001.

Gofman J, *Preventing Breast Cancer: The Story of a Major, Proven, Preventable Cause of this Disease*, CNR Book Division, Committee for Nuclear Responsibility Inc, USA 1996.

Gray J, *State of the Evidence: The Connection Between Breast Cancer and the Environment*, The Breast Cancer Fund, USA 2008.

Gray J, *State of the Evidence: The Connection Between Breast Cancer and the Environment*, The Breast Cancer Fund, USA 2010.

Hardy D, Hardy M, Killick M, Killick K, *Pyramid Energy: The Philosophy of God, The Science of Man*, Cadaka Industries & Copple House, 1987 USA.

Havas M, *Dirty Eectricity: An invisible pollutant in schools*, Environmental Resource Studies Trent University, Ontario, Canada 2006.

Havas M, Electrical Pollution Taskforce. Markham, Environmental Resource Studies Trent University, Ontario, Canada 2005.

Havas M, *Power quality affects teacher wellbeing and student behavior in three Minnesota schools*, ScienceDirect Elsevier, USA 2008.

Henshaw DL, *What about the effect of EMFs on melatonin and breast cancer? A set of frequently asked questions specifically about melatonin*, Bristol University, UK 2006.

Johansson O, *The Effects of Radiation in the Cause of Cancer, Icon*, issue 4, 2005.

Kane RC, *Cellphone Telephone Russian Roulette*, Vantage Press, USA 2001.

Labi S, *Unlocking the riddles of a condition that prefers to keep secrets*. Article published in online journal *Nature* and reported in *The Sunday Telegraph*, 3 May 2009.

Lantz S, *Chemical Free Kids: Raising Children in a Toxic World*, Joshua Books, Australia 2009.

Lew Lim T, *Biostimulation Mechanism with Intranasal Light Therapy – What really happens under the surface*, MedicLights Research Inc, Canada 2011.

Lew Lim T, *Intranasal Light Therapy bridges Traditional Chinese Medicine with Modern Medicine*, Mediclights Research Inc, Canada 2012.

Liberman J, MD PhD, *Light: Medicine of the Future*, Bear & Company, USA 1991.

Lister S, *NHS accused over women's breast cancer screening risks*, The Times, UK 2009.

Lynes B, *Rife's World of Electromedicine: The Story, the Corruption and the Promise*, USA 2009.

Maret K, *Electromagnetic fields and human health*. International Conference Electromagnetic Fields and Human Health, Kazakhstan, September 2003.

Maret K, *Sickness rate of workers in electrolysis sections of titanic – magnesium and zinc industries of the Republic of Kazakhstan*. International conference Electromagnetic Fields and Human Health, Kazakhstan, September 2003.

Medical Tactile Imaging, SureTouch Visual Mapping System, *Digital Breast Exam Breakthrough: New technology for the early detection of breast cancer*, USA 2002.

Meyl K, *Cellullar Communication by Magnetic Scalar Waves*, Progress in Electromagnetics Research Symposium Proceedings, Moscow, Russia, Aug 19-23 2012.

Meyl K, *Scalar Wave Transponder*, third edition, INDEL GmbH publishing department, Villingen-Schwenningen, Germany 2011.

Milham S, *Dirty Electricity: Electrification and The Diseases of Civilization*, iUniverse Inc, USA 2010.

Milham S, *Evidence that dirty electricity is causing the worldwide epidemics of obesity and diabetes*, Electromagn Biol Med, Early Online: 1-4 Informa Healthcare USA, Inc. doi: 10.3109/15368378.2013.783853.

Milham S, *Historical evidence that electrification caused the 20th century epidemic of 'diseases of civilization'*, Elsevier Ltd, 2009 doi: 10.1016/j.mehy.2009.09.032.

Milham S, Morgan LL, *A New Electromagnetic Exposure Metric: High Frequency Voltage Transients Associated with Increased Cancer Incidence in Teachers in a California School*, Am J Ind Med 2008, Wiley-Liss 2008.

Milham S, Stetzer D, *Dirty Electricity, Chronic Stress, Neurotransmitters and Disease*, 2013, www.sammilham.com

Morgan G, Ward R, Barton M, *The contribution of cytotoxic chemotherapy to survival in adult malignancies*, Department of Radiation Oncology, Northern Sydney Cancer Centre, Royal North Shore Hospital, NSW, AUS 2004.

Meyers BA, *PEMF: The 5th Element of Health*, Balboa Press, USA 2013.

Myss C PhD, *Anatomy of the Spirit: The Seven Stages of Power and Healing*, Bantam AUS and NZ 1997.

Neophytou C MD, *Encyclopedia of the Mind, Body & Spirit*, Lindlahr Publishing, AUS 1996.

Ober C, Sinatra S MD, Zucker M, *Earthing: The most important health discovery ever?*, Basic Health Publications Inc, USA 2010.

O'Neill JJ, *Prodigal Genius: The Life of Nikola Tesla*, Ives Washburn, USA 1944.

Oschman JL, Prof, *Energy Medicine The Scientific Basis*, Churchill Livingstone, UK 2000.

Rees C, Havas M, Public Health SOS: *The Shadow Side of the Wireless Revolution: 110 Questions on Electromagnetic Pollution*, Commonwealth Club of California forum, Wide Angle Health LLC, USA 2008.

Roy R, *Science of Whole Person Healing – Proceedings of the First Interdisciplinary International Conference*, iUniverse Inc, USA 2003.

Shealy CN PhD, Myss CM PhD, *The Ring of Fire and DHEA: A Theory for Energetic Restoration of Adrenal Reserves, Subtle Energies*, Vol 6 No 2, 1995.

Slesin L, *Faulty DNA repair may explain EMF role in childhood leukemia, Microwavenews*, vol XXVIII, no 10, December 2008.

Stevens RG, Wilson BW, Anderson LE, (eds), *The Melatonin Hypothesis: Breast Cancer and the Use of Electric Power*, Columbus Battelle Press, USA 1997.

The National Foundation for Alternative Medicine USA, *The Health Effects of Electrical Pollution*, The National Foundation for Alternative Medicine, USA.

Valentina N, *Occupational and opulation health risks of radio frequency electromagnetic fields*, Electromagnetic Fields and Human Health report, Kazakhstan 2003.

Walsh WJ, PhD, *Nutrient Power: Heal Your BioChemistry and Heal Your Brain*, Skyhorse Publishing, 2012 USA

World Health Organization, *Extremely Low Frequency Fields*, Published under the joint sponsorship of the International Labour Organization, the International Commission on Non-Ionizing Radiation Protection, and the World Health Organization Environmental Health Criteria 238, 2007.

Zharkinov E, *Sickness rate of workers in electrolysis sections of titanic-magnesium and zinc industries of Kazakhstan report*, Electromagnetic Fields and Human Health conference, Kazakhstan 2003.

WEBSITES AND ONLINE RESOURCES INCLUDED IN RESEARCH

www.abc.net.au/news/stories/2008/11/25/2429401.htm

www.businessinsurance.com/apps/pbcs.dll/article?AID

www.buergerwelle.de/pdf/la_quinta_cancer_cluster.pdf

www.dirtyelectricity.ca/images/08_HavasOlstad_schools1.pdf

www.ecopolitan.com/health-resources/emfprotection/147-health-effects-radio

www.emfacts.com

www.electricalpollution.com.documents/08_Havas_UFL_SCENIHR.pdf

www.electricpollution.com/Lloyd_Morganexcerpts.htm

www.emfsolutions.ca/compact_fluorescent_bulbs_are_dangerous.htm

www.emrpolicy.org/public_policy/schools/magda_havas_hsn_presentation.pdf

www.europarl.europa.eu/sides/getDoc.do?pubRef

www.icems.eu

http://journals.sfu.ca/seemj/index.php/seemj/article/viewFile/200/164

www.jerseymastconcern.co.uk

www.mediclights.com

www.nasa.gov/topics/nasalaife/features/heals.html.

www.nextup.org

www.ovantis.co.uk/introscan.html

www.stop-emf.ca/stopinfo/HavasPresentationTaskForce.pdf

techtran.msfc.nasa.gov/support/images/MFS-31651-1_TreatmentOral
Mucostitis.pdf

www.thehealinguniverse.com

www.virtualmedicinehealth.net

NOTES

PART 1: LIGHT THAT HARMS

CHAPTER 1

1. Milham S, *Historical evidence that electrification caused the 20th century epidemic of 'diseases of civilisation'*, Medical Hypotheses 74 (2010) 337-345 doi: 10.1016/j.mehy.2009.08.032.

2. Elwardt HA ND PhD, *Let's Stop the #1 Killer of Americans Today – A Natural Approach to Preventing & Reversing Heart Disease*, USA. Note: Heart attacks are just one type of cardiovascular disease. Included in cardiovascular disease are: Atherosclerosis, Coronary Artery Disease (CAD), Sudden Cardiac Death (SCD), Congestive Heart Failure, Heart Valve Disease, Congenital Heart Disease, Heart Muscle Disease, (Cardiomyopathy) Pericardial Disease, Aortic Aneurysm, Marfan Syndrome, Carotid Artery Disease, Vascular Disease, Peripheral Artery Disease (PAD), Renal Artery Disease, Raynaud's Disease, Bueger's Disease, Peripheral Venous Disease, Varicose Veins, Deep Vein Thrombosis (DVT), Pulmonary Embolism and Stroke.

3. Chadna SL, Gopinath N, Shekhawat S, *Urban-rural difference in the prevalence of coronary heart disease and its risk factors*, Bull World Health Org 1997;75(1):31-8.

4. Milham S, Ossiander EM, *Historical evidence that residential electrification caused the emergence of the childhood leukemia peak*, Medical Hypotheses (2001) 56(3), 290-295 doi: 10.1054/mehy.2000.1138.

5. Milham S, *Historical evidence that electrification caused the 20th century epidemic of 'diseases of civilisation'*, Medical Hypotheses 74 (2010) 337-345 doi: 10.1016/j.mehy.2009.08.032.

6. Struewing J, Abeliovich D, Peretz T et al, 1995, *The carrier frequency of the BRCA1 185DELag mutations in approximately 1 percent in Ashkenazi Jewish individuals*, Nt Genet 11:198 200 Neuhausen S, Gilewski T, Norton L et al 1996, *Recurrent BRCA2 6174delT mutations in Ashkenazi Jewish women affected by breast cancer*, Nat Genet 13:126-128 Tonin P, Weber B, Offit K et al 1996, *Frequency of recurrent BRCA1 and BRCA2 mutations in Ashkenazi Jewish breast cancer families*, Nat Med 2:1179-1183.

7. Westman et al, 2010, *Low cancer incidence rates in Ohio Amish Cancer Causes Control*, doi 10.1007/S10552-009-9435-7.192 193.

8. Shuldiner and Sorkin, 2003.

9. Hamman RF, Barancik JJ, Lilienfeld AM, *Patterns of mortality in the Old Order Amish, Am J Epidemiol* 1981;114(6):345–61.

10. Katz M, Ferketich A, Harley A *et al*, 2000, *Cancer screening among Amish adults*, In: '29th Annual Meeting of the American Society of Preventive Oncology, 2005, San Francisco, California USA.

11. Holder J and Warren AC, 1998, *Prevalance of Alzheimer's disease and apolipoprotein E allele frequencies in the Old Order Amish, J Neuropsychiatry Clin Neurosci.* 10 1:100-102.

12. Ruff ME, 2005, *Attention deficit disorder and stimulant use: an epidemic of modernity, Clin Pediatr* (Philadelphia) 44:557-563.

13. Dirty electricity is caused by arcing, sparking and anything that interrupts current flow, especially modern switching power supplies. Thomas Edison complained that his original "Jumbo" generators had serious commutator brush arcing so dirty electricity has been here since the electric grid was established. Early electric generating equipment and electric motors used commutators, carbon brushes and split rings that would inject high frequency voltage transients into the 50/60 Hz electricity being generated and distributed.

14. The initial fight or flight reaction causes increased sympathetic nervous system activity and the adrenal glands release epinephrine and norepinephrine into the bloodstream. The adrenal glands also release corticosteroid hormones. Digestion stops, blood pressure and pulse rate increase and the heart pumps more blood to the muscles. Blood sugar levels increase. If stress is chronic, epinephrine and norepinephrine levels decline but corticosteroid secretion continues at above-normal levels. Chronic disturbance of the catecholamine system inevitably results in disease. Milham's words in Milham S, Stetzer D, *Dirty Electricity, Chronic Stress, Neurotransmitters and Disease*, 2013, www.sammilham.com

15. Milham S, Stetzer D, *Dirty Electricity, Chronic Stress, Neurotransmitters and Disease*, 2013, www.sammilham.com

16. Milham S, Stetzer D, *Dirty Electricity, Chronic Stress, Neurotransmitters and Disease*, 2013, www.sammilham.com

17. Coghill R, p 84.

18. Full decision at: http://www.austlii.edu.au/au/cases/cth/aat/2013/105.html

CHAPTER 2

1. Genuis SJ, p 8.

2. Juutilainen J, Kumlin T, Naarala, J, 2006 *Do extremely low frequency magnetic*

fields enhance the effects of environmental carcinogens? A meta-analysis of experimental studies, Int J Radiat Biol 82:1-12. *In vitro* and short-term animal studies. Juutilainen *et al.* found the majority of studies reviewed were positive, suggesting that magnetic fields do interact with other chemical and physical exposures. The percentage of the 65 studies with positive effects was highest when the EMF exposure preceded the other exposure. The review collected 65 studies published between 1986 and 2002. The Juutilainen *et al.* 2006 study revealed that: the combined effects of toxic agents and ELF magnetic fields together enhances damage as compared to the toxic exposure alone, and the radical pair mechanism (oxidative damage due to free radicals) is cited as a good candidate to explain these results.

3. Lai and Singh were the first to report this effect (1996-1997). Phillips *et al*, O'Neill, Svendenstal, Rudiger, Schar amongst others. Refer: *Microwave News, European Labs Show EMFs Induce DNA Breaks: Intermittent, Not Continuous, Fields Are Effective* Vol XX11 No 5 Sept/Oct 2002, *Microwave News, Radiation Research and the Cult of Negative Studies* July 31, 2006, *Microwave News, Science Gets It Wrong on DNA Breaks* September 3, 2008, *Microwave News, Faulty DNA Repair May Explain EMF Role in Childhood Leukemia* Dec 15, 2008.

4. *Microwave News, Finns See RF-Chemical Synergy* March 3, 2009 – refer *Enhancement of chemically induced reactive oxygen species production and DNA damage in human SH-SY5Y neuroblastoma cells by 872 MHz radiofrequency radiation, Mutat Res*: 2009 Mar 9;662 (1-2):54-8. doi:10.1016/j.mrfmmm.2008.12.005. Epub 2008 Dec 24, *PubMed* – indexed for MEDLINE PMID: 19135463.

5. The private and confidential advice from law firm Watson and Renner, Washington DC to the electrical utilities worldwide.

6. *Electromagnetic fields and public health: extremely low frequency fields and cancer,* Fact sheet No 263, WHO, October 2001.

7. *Electromagnetic fields and public health: exposure to extremely low frequency fields,* Fact sheet No 322, WHO, June 2007.

8. Genuis SJ, p 8.

9. Becker R, p 215.

10. Lantz S, p 43.

11. The sanitary norms address the 1–400 kHz frequency. By order of the Head State Sanitary Physician of the Republic of Kazakhstan, 28 Nov 2003, r.No 69.

12. (For environmental reasons). Ontario Hydro Power Quality Reference Guide – Mitigation Techniques – Page 83 recommends the installation of filters to control harmonics. The IEEE (Institute of Electrical and Electronics Engineers) Recommended Practices and Requirements for Harmonic Control in

Electrical Power Systems IEEE 519-1992. Through its highly cited publications, conferences, technology standards and professional and educational activities, IEEE is the trusted voice on a wide variety of areas ranging from aerospace systems, computers and telecommunications to biomedical engineering, electric power and consumer electronics.

13. Full decision at: http://www.austlii.edu.au/au/cases/cth/aat/2013/105.html

CHAPTER 3

1. Armstrong B et al, 1994, *Association between exposure to pulsed electromagnetic fields and cancer in electric utility workers in Quebec, Canada and France, Am J of Epidemiol* 140, (9): 805-820.

2. Milham S, p 59.

3. Milham S, p 67.

4. Author's discussions with Dr Milham.

5. Milham S, p 92.

6. Reynolds *et al.* 1999.

CHAPTER 4

1. Technical papers provide a solid electrical and biomolecular basis for these effects. A recent paper by Ozen showed that transients induce much stronger current density levels in the human body than does the powerline 60Hz signal. Another technical paper discusses the authors' findings that high frequency communication signals on powerlines also induce much stronger electrical currents in the human body than a low frequency signal of the same strength. The induced currents disturb normal intercellular communications. Refer: Ozen S, 2007 *Low-frequency Transient Electric and Magnetic Fields Coupling to Child Body, Radiation Protection Dosimetry* (2007), pp 1-6; and Vignati M, and Giuliani L, 1997 *Radiofrequency exposure near high-voltage lines* Environ Health Perspect 105 (Suppl6):1569-1573 (1997).

2. At the September 2003 international conference which preceded Kazakhstan's move to issue sanitary norms (November 2003) to protect their citizens.

3. Maret K, p 5.

4. Havas M, Olstad A, p 1-2. Currently available for viewing at: www.dirtyelectricity.ca/images/08_HavasOlstad_schools1.pdf

5. Milham S, p 58.

6. In addition to causing health problems directly, this high-frequency pollution also leads to another source of problems: ground currents. Further reading

on this subject is available: *Relationship of Electric Power Quality to Milk Production of Dairy Herds*, Hillman D, Stetzer D, Graham M, Goeke CL, Mathson K, VanHorn HH, Wilcox CJ.

7. *Extremely Low Frequency Fields,* published under the joint sponsorship of the International Labour Organization, the International Commission on Non-Ionizing Radiation Protection, and the World Health Organization Environmental Health Criteria 238, p 11. WHO 2007.

CHAPTER 5

1. Valentina N, p 14.

2. Santini 2001, *La Presse Medicale.*

3. Gunter M, Strickler H, and colleagues at the Albert Einstein College of Medicine, New York.

4. Havas M, Olstad A, pp 1-2.

5. Milham S, p 80. Milham, S, *Evidence that dirty electricity is causing the worldwide epidemics of obesity and diabetes, Electromagn Biol Med*, Early Online: 1-4 Informa Healthcare USA, Inc. doi: 10.3109/15368378.2013.783853.

6. Further information: The French zone is the Conservatoire Naturel des Espaces Naturels Rhône-Alpes. The Italian zone is within the Vena del Gesso Regional Park near the town of Brisighella in the province of Ravenna. This electrosmog-free B&B is 2.5km from the station of Brisighella (Faenza-Florence line, not electrified) and is in the middle of an unspoilt landscape just next to the Refuge Zone. B&B "Eremodellupo" Associazione Italiana Elettrosensibili –A.I.E. –Via Cadorna, 5, 35123 Padova (PD) tel: 02/6431425 – www.elettrosensibili.it presidente@elettrosensibili.it Source: Next-up Organization, Next-Up News Nr 1391 Creation of the first free EHS zone in Italy, August 21, 2010.

7. Havas M, *Diabetes and Electromagnetic Fields: the evidence*, Next-Up Organization.

8. Havas M, *Electromagnetic Biology and Medicine*, 25:259, 2007.

CHAPTER 6

1. Gofman J, p 4 & Wanebo CK, and colleagues following on from McKenzie I, 1965.

2. Wertheimer N, Leeper E, *Adult cancer related to electrical wires near the home, Int J Epidemiol*, 1982 11:345–355.

3. Erren T in Stevens RG, Wilson BW, Anderson LE, p 731.

4. Jing-Wen Sun *et al. Electromagnetic Field Exposure and Male Breast Cancer Risk: A Meta-analysis of 18 Studies, Asian Pacific Journal of Cancer Prevention* Vol 14 2013 1, 523-528.

5. A handful of other cancers, including ovarian and salivary gland cancers, were also reported. Louis Slesin www.microwavenews.com

6. Henshaw D, p 6.

7. Gray J, 2008, p 6.

8. Lister S.

9. Evans N, 2004 p 4.

10. Gray J, 2010 p 62. 196 197

11. Gray J, 2010 p 63.

12. The BioInitiative Report, 2007.

13. Gray J, 2010, p 60. Referenced from: Kloog I, Haim A, Stevens RG, Barchana M, Portnov BA, 2008, *Chronobiol Int*, 25:65-8.

14. Dr David Blask at the American Association for Cancer Research, 2003.

CHAPTER 7

1. Havas M, *Study finds Vatican Radio Causes Cancer,* July 30, 2010 – www.magdahavas.com

2. Milham S, p 86.

3. Lester JR, and Moore DF 1982 *Cancer Mortality and Air Force Bases* Journal of Bioelectricity 1 (1): 72-82 – www.magdahavas.com

4. Davis RL, Mostofi FK, *Cluster of testicular cancer in police officers exposed to hand-held radar,* Am J Ind Med 1993; 24 (2):231–3. [26].

5. *Laptops on the Legs Affect Male Fertility* – www.magdahavas.com

6. Hallberg O, Johansson O, pp 3-8.

7. Hallberg O, Johansson O, p 3.

8. O'Connor E, *Why people are worried about EMF: A UK perspective,* UK Radiation Research Trust Workshop on EMF and Health: Science and Policy, European Commission, Brussels, 11-12 February 2009.

9. Levitt BB, Lai H, *Biological effects from exposure to electromagnetic radiation emitted by cell tower base stations and other antenna arrays, Environmental Reviews* 18:369-395A, Journal of the National Research Council Canada.

10. Judgement of the Crown Court of Nanterre France, February 4, 2009.

11. Judgement of The Tribunal de Grande Instance (District Court) of Carpentras France, February 16, 2009.

12. Further information at: www.europarl.europa.eu sides/getDoc.do?pubRef

13. The BBB is the same in a rat as it is in a human being.

14. Johansson O in Firstenberg A, page 5.

15. Kane RC, p 102. Lai H and Singh NP, *Acute Low-Intensity Microwave Exposure Increases DNA Single-Strand Breaks in Rat Brain Cells in press Microwaves Break DNA in Brain: Cellular Phone Industry Skeptical,* Microwave News 14, No 6, November-December 1994, Lai H and Singh NP, *International Journal of Rad.* Biology 69 (1996):513-21.

16. Morgan LL, lead author of the report last August *Cellphones and Brain Tumors: 15 Reasons for Concern, Science, Spin and the Truth Behind Interphone* – www.electromagnetichealth.org electromagnetic-health-blog/confused-by-the-media-coverage-of-the-inter- phone-brain-tumor-study

17. Hardell L, Carlberg M, Söderqvist F, Mild KH, *Case Control Study of the association between malignant brain tumours diagnosed between 2007 and 2009 and mobile and cordless phone use,* International Journal of Oncology, Vol 43 issue 6 doi: 10.3892/ijo.2013.2111, pp 1833-1845.

18. Hardell L, Carlberg M, *Using the Hill viewpoints from 1965 for evaluating strengths of evidence of the risk for brain tumors associated with use of mobile and cordless phone,* DOI 10.1515/reveh-2013-0006, *Rev Environ Health,* 28(2-3): 97–106.

19. West JG, Kapoor, NS, Liao S-Y, Chen JW, Bailey L, Nagourney RA, *Multifocal Breast Cancer in Young Women with Prolonged Contact between Their Breasts and Their Cellular Phones Case, Reports in Medicine* vol 2013, Article ID 354682, 5 pages 2013 dx.doi.org/10.1155/2013/354682.

20. *Children and mobile phones: The health of the following generations is in danger,* Russian National Committee on Non-Ionizing Radiation Protection Moscow, Russia, April 14, 2008.

21. Electromagnetic Biology and Medicine (2013 Jun; 32(2):200-208) Informa UK Ltd.

22. *Digital Portable Phones Affect the Heart* – www.magdahavas.com

23. www.scribd.com/doc/27618514/CEM-Sentenza-Corte-d-Appello-Di-Brescia

24. *Living with EHS in an Electrified Wireless World,* Rewire Me eMagazine p 20.

25. Vogel G, *Next Asbestos Could Be In Air, Business Insurance,* September 13, 2010

26. Articles written by Havas M, November 26, 2010 – www.magdahavas.com

27. Stever H, Kuhn J, Otten C, Wunder B, Harst W *Verhaltensanderung unter elektromagnetischer Exposition* Pilotstudie. Institut für Mathematik. Arbeitsgruppe. Bildungsinformatik Universität Koblenz-Landau; 2005 – www. agbi.uni-landau.de/ materailien.htm. Source: #664 DECT and Bee Decline, March 3, 2007 – www.emfacts.com

A series of studies by Wolfgang Harst, Jochen Kuhn and Hermann Stever at Landau University in Germany, demonstrated the effect of pulsed, digital radiation. In their study, two beehives were unexposed and two beehives were exposed to a cordless DECT phone. Twenty-five bees were selected from each hive and released 800 metres away. In the unexposed hives 16 and 17 bees returned in 28 and 32 minutes respectively. In the DECT-exposed hives 6 bees returned to one in 38 minutes, and none returned to the other hive at all. In the exposed hives, there were 21 percent fewer cells constructed in the hive frames after nine days.

28. *Nature* Vol 429, pp 177-180, May 13, 2004.

   In reporting that EMF disrupt crypto-chrome-based magnetic navigation, Goldsworthy states that Thorsten Ritz and his co-workers showed that even weak electromagnetic radiation over a wide range of radio frequencies completely prevented robins orienting for navigation in a steady magnetic field simulating that of the Earth, the same is probably true for bees.

29. Yoshii and co-workers 2009.

30. Press Release *IARC classifies radiofrequency electromagnetic fields as possibly carcinogenic to humans,* WHO IARC May 31, 2011 – www.iarc.fr/en/media-centre/pr/2011/pdfs/pr208_E.pdf

31. *Free fiber for Swiss Schools WiFi warnings* – www.magdahavas.com

32. *Effects of modulated VHF fields on the central nervous system,* Ann NY Acad Sci 247: 74-81.

33. ISBN 10 3-540-32717-7, Springer 2006.

34. Excerpted from: *The potential dangers of electromagnetic fields and their effect on the environment* Parliamentary Assembly – Council of Europe Report. Committee on the Environment, Agriculture and Local and Regional Affairs Rapporteur: Mr Jean Huss, Luxembourg, Socialist Group.

   Document 12608, Points 58-61 – http://assemly.coe.int

   Recommendations were adopted by Parliamentary Assembly of the Council of Europe, May 27, 2011, Resolution 1815.

CHAPTER 8

1. Herbert M PhD MD, Sage C MA, *Findings in Autism (ASD) Consistent with Electromagnetic Fields (EMF) and Radiofrequency Radiation (RFR),* The BioInitiative Report 2012 Section 20.

2. Ang ESBC, Gluncic V, Duque A, Schafer ME, Rakic P (2006) *Prenatal exposure to ultrasound waves impacts neuronal migration in mice,* Proceedings of the National Academy of Science 103(34):12903-12910.

3. McDonald ME, Paul JF, *Timing of Increased Autistic Disorder Cumulative Incidence* National Health and Environmental Effects Research Laboratory, US Environmental Protection Agency. Environ.Sci.Technol. 2010,44,2112-2118.

4. Becker R, p 260.

5. Journal of the Australasian College of Nutritional and Environmental Medicine, November 2007, Vol 26, No 2, pp 3-7.

6. Maret K, p 9.

7. Excerpts from transcript: Dr George Carlo's meeting with Scrutiny Panel Jersey Mast Concern, UK.

8. transcripts.cnn.com/transcripts/0904/03/lkl.01.html

9. Eisenstein M, p 68. Refer: Noble GR, *et al. Acellular and whole cell pertussis vaccines in Japan* reports of a visit by US scientists. *Journal of the America Medical Association* 1987; 257:1351-56. Scott J, *Report: US slips in fight to cut infant mortality, Press & Sun Bulletin* (extracted from the *Los Angeles Times*, March 1, 1990). Cherry JD *et al. Report of the task force on pertussis and pertussis immunization, Pediatr* (Jun 1988); 81 (6): 933-84.

10. Genuis SJ, p 3.

11. Lintas C, Sacco R, Persico AM, *Genome-wide expression studies in autism spectrum disorder, Rett syndrome and Down syndrome, Neurobiol* Dis 45 (1):57-68.

12. Herbert M PhD MD, Sage C MA, *Findings in Autism (ASD) Consistent with Electromagnetic Fields (EMF) and Radiofrequency Radiation (RFR),* The BioInitiative Report 2012, Section 20.

13. Gupta, 1988.

14. Sparks and Hunsaker, 1988.

15. Sturner *et al*, 1994.

16. Genuis SJ, p 5.

17. Stevens RG, Wilson BW, Anderson LE, p 40-41. The pineal gland secretes the neuroendocrine hormone melatonin that is synthesized from the neurotransmitter serotonin.

18. University of Texas Health Science Center at San Antonio *Serotonin Plays Role in Many Autism Cases, Studies Confirm,* February 24, 2011. Retrieved December 19, 2013 from: www.sciencedaily.com/releases/2011/02/110224121940.htm

19. Harrington RA *et al, Serotonin Hypothesis of Autism: Implications for Selective Serotonin Reuptake Use During Pregnancy, Autism* Res 2013, 6:149-168 doi: 10.1002/aur.1288 International Society for Autism Research, Wiley Periodicals, Inc.

20. Rees C, Havas M, p 22.

21. Rees C, Havas M, p 65.

22. Source: #821 Autism and DECT Baby Monitors, November 23, 2007
www.emfacts.com

23. Havas M, *Are DECT baby monitors dangerous?*, November 7, 2010
– www.magdahavas.com

24. Kane RC PhD, *A Possible Association between Fetal/neonatal Exposure to Radiofrequency Electromagnetic Radiation and the Increased Incidence of Autism Spectrum Disorders (ASD)*, Medical Hypotheses (2004) 62, 195-197.

References referred to in Kane's article are below:

1. Berman E, Kinn JB, and Carter HB, *Observations of mouse fetuses after irradiation with 2.45 GHz microwaves*, Health Physics 35, pp 791-801, 1978.

2. Kaplan J, Polson P, Rebert C, Lunan K, and Gage M, *Biological and behavioral effects of prenatal and postnatal exposure to 2450-MHz electromagnetic radiation in the squirrel monkey*, Radio Science 17(5S), pp 135S-144S, 1982.

3. Sagripanti JL, and Swicord ML, *DNA structural changes caused by microwave radiation*, Int J Radiat Biol 50(1), pp 47-50, 1986.

4. Leszczynski D, Joenväärä S, Reivinen J, and Kuokka R. *Non-thermal activation of the hsp27/p38MAPK stress pathway by mobile phone radiation in human endothelial cells: Molecular mechanism for cancer and blood-brain barrier-related effects*, Differentiation 70, pp 120-129, 2002.

5. Sagripanti JL, Swicord ML, and Davis CC, *Microwave effects on plasmid DNA*, Radiation Research 110, pp 219-231, 1987.

6. Fucic A, Garaj-Vrhovac V, Skara M, and Dimitrovic B, *X-rays, microwaves and vinyl chloride monomer: their clastogenic and aneugenic activity, using the micronucleus assay on human lymphocytes*, Mutat Res 282(4), pp 265-271, 1992.

7. Maes A, Verschaeve L, Arroyo A, De Wagter C, and Vercruyssen L, *In vitro cytogenetic effects of 2450 MHz waves on human peripheral blood lymphocytes*, Bioelectromagnetics 14(6), pp 495-501, 1993.

8. Sarkar S, Ali S, and Behari J, *Effect of low power microwave on the mouse genome: a direct DNA analysis*, Mutat Res 320 (1-2), pp 141-147, 1994.

9. Lai H, and Singh NP, *Acute low-intensity microwave exposure increases DNA single-strand breaks in rat brain cells*, Bioelectromagnetics, 16(3) pp 207-210, 1995.

10. Lai H, and Singh NP, *Single- and double-strand DNA breaks in rat brain cells after acute exposure to radiofrequency electromagnetic radiation*, Int J Radiat Biol 69(4), pp 513-521, 1996.

11. Repacholi MH, Basten A, Gebski V, Noonan D, Finnie J, and Harris AW, *Lymphomas in E mu-Pim1 transgenic mice exposed to pulsed 900 MHz electromagnetic fields, Radiat Res* 147(5), pp 631-640, 1997.

12. Phillips JL, Ivaschuk O, Ishida-Jones T, Jones RA, Campbell-Beachler M, and Haggren W, *DNA damage in Molt-4 T-lymphoblastoid cells exposed to cellular telephone radiofrequency fields in vitro, Bioelectrochemistry and Bioenergetics* 45, pp 103-110, 1998.

13. Hardell L, Hansson Mild K, Pahlson A, Hallquist A, *Ionizing radiation, cellular telephones and the risk of brain tumors, Europ J Cancer Prevent* 10, pp 523-529, 2001.

14. Byrd RS, Sigman M, Bono M, *et al, Report to the legislature on the principal findings from the epidemiology of autism in California: a comprehensive pilot study,* M.I.N.D. Institute, University of California, Davis, 2002.

15. Bawin SM, Kaczmarek LK, and Adey WR, *Effects of modulated VHF fields on the central nervous system,* Ann NY Acad. Sci 247, pp 74-81,1975.

16. Chiang H, Yao GD, Fang QS, Wang KQ, Lu DZ, Zhou YK, *Health effects of environmental electromagnetic fields, J Bioelectricity* 8:127-131 1989.

17. Lai H, Horita A, and Guy AW, *Microwave irradiation affects radial-arm maze performance in the rat, Bioelectromagnetics* 15(2), pp 95-104, 1994.

18. von Klitzing L, *Low-frequency pulsed electromagnetic fields influence EEG of man, Phys. Medica* 11, pp 77-80, 1995.

19. Salford LG, Brun A, Sturesson K, Eberhardt JL, and Persson BR, *Permeability of the blood-brain radiation on cytolytic T lymphocytes, FASEB J* 10(8), pp 913-919, 1996.

20. Paul Raj R, Behari J, and Rao AR, *Effect of amplitude modulated RF radiation on calcium ion efflux and ODC activity in chronically exposed rat brain, Indian J Biochem Biophys* 36(5), pp 337-340, 1999.

21. Cleary SF, Du Z, Cao G, Liu LM, and McCrady C, *Effect of isothermal radiofrequency barrier induced by 915 MHz electromagnetic radiation, continuous wave and modulated at 8, 16, 50, and 200 Hz, Microsc Res Tech* 27(6), pp 535-542, 1994.

22. d'Ambrosio G, Massa R, Scarfi MR, and Zeni O, *Cytogenetic damage in human lymphocytes following GMSK phase modulated microwave exposure, Bioelectromagnetics* 23, pp 7-13, 2002.

23. Persson BR, Salford LG, and Brun A, *Blood-brain barrier permeability in rats exposed to electromagnetic fields used in wireless communication,* Wireless Network 3, pp 455-461, 1997.

24. Bertrand J, Mars A, Boyle C, Bove F, Yeargin-Allsopp M, Decoufle P, *Prevalence*

of Autism in a United States Population: The Brick Township, New Jersey Investigation, Pediatrics 108 (5), pp 1155-1161, Nov 2001.

25. Taylor B, Miller E, Farringdon *et al, MMR Vaccine and Autism: No Epidemiological Evidence for a Causal Association, The Lancet* 353, pp 2026-2029, 1999.

26. Chakrabarti S, & Fombonne E, *Pervasive Developmental Disorders in Preschool Children, JAMA* 285 (24), 2001. Source: www.latitudes.org/articles/electrical_sensitivity_articles.html#A Possible Association.

CHAPTER 9

1. Lichtenstein P, Holm NV, Verkasalo PK, Iliadou A, Kaprio J, Koskenvuo M *et al. Environmental and heritable factors in the causation of cancer: Analyses of cohorts of twins from Sweden, Denmark and Finland, N Engl J Med* 2000:343:78-85.

2. Van-Steensil Moll *et al,* 1985, Infante-Rivard, 1995.

3. Nordstrom S, Birke E, Gustavsson L, *Reproductive hazards among workers at high voltage substations. Bioelectromagnetics* 1983; 4:91-101. Nordenson I, Hansoon MK, Nordstrom S, Sweins A, Birke E, *Clastogenic effects in human lymphocytes of power frequency electric fields: in vivo and in vitro studies, Radiat Environ Biophys* 202 203.

4. Spitz MR, Cole CC, *Reports significant increase in incidence of brain tumors among children of fathers occupationally exposed to electromagnetic fields, Am J of Epidemiol* 1211985:924. Wilkins 3rd, JR, Koutras RA. *Paternal occupation and brain cancer in offspring: a mortality-based case-control study, Am J Ind Med* 1988; 14:299-318. Johnson CC, Spitz MR *Childhood nervous system tumors: an assessment of risk associated with paternal occupations involving use, repair or manufacture of electrical and electronic equipment, Int J Epidemiol* 1989, 18:756-62.

5. Shen *et al,* Leukemia & Lymphoma 2008.

6. This polymorphism/snp is known by a variety of designations: 'Ex9+16G>A' and 'Arg280His'.

7. Research of Juan Manuel Mejia-Arangure.

8. Slesin L, p 1.

9. Hallberg and Johansson report that deaths due to asbestosis were not known until after the 1960s despite the fact that asbestos has been used as a building material since the end of the 19th century.

10. Additional research in Johansson O, 2005.

11. Firstenberg A, para 25.

12. Hallberg and Johansson, 2002B, 2004, 2005a.

13. This is taken directly from The BioInitiative Report *Summary for the Public.* Further reading is available in Section 12 of the report.

14. From an article published in *American Journal of Epidemiology,* Nov 2008.

15. Frolich H, 1978. Oschman JL, p 135.

16. Alteration of the plateau phase of calcium signalling implicates the calcium channel as a site of field interaction. Liburdy RP, *Calcium signaling in lymphocytes and ELF fields – Evidence for an electric field metric and a site of interaction involving the calcium ion channel. Separate studies of lymphocytes stimulated with a mitogen showed that a weak 3 Hz pulsed magnetic field sharply reduced calcium influx, while a 60 Hz signal, under identical conditions increased calcium influx (Adey R, 1996).* Volume 301, Issue 1, 13 April 1992, Pages 53-59, DOI: 10.1016/0014-5793(92)80209-Y. Oschman JL, p.252

    The 2001 court-case referred to in my book, *Silent Fields The Growing Cancer Cluster Story: When Electricity Kills,* brought attention to a study that discovered a fundamental calcium ion resonance in the vicinity of 50 Hz.

17. Oschman JL, p 96, Dr Robert O Becker contended that the pulsing DC electrical system (brain waves) set the tone of the entire nervous system.

18. Oschman JL, p 97

19. Oschman JL, p 96, Dr Robert O Becker contended that the pulsing DC electrical system (brain waves) set the tone of the entire nervous system.

20. Excerpted and summarized from: *The Health Effects of Electromagnetic Fields,* Dr Martin Blank November 18, 2010, Commonwealth Club of California program and Mercola J MD, *Caution: This Common Device Can Double Your Risk of Getting a Brain Tumor,* January 19, 2011. The highly respected Dr Martin Blank PhD is an associate professor at Columbia University in the Department of Physiology and Cellular Bophysics and a researcher in Bioelectromagnetics. Blank authored the section on stress proteins for The Bioinitiative Report and edited the journal *Pathology*'s Special Issue *on the Biological Effects of Electromagnetic Fields.* Blank is also past president of the Bioelectromagnetics Society, has two PhD's, one from Columbia University in Physical Chemistry, and another from Cambridge University in Colloid Science (biology, physics and chemistry).

21. *Public Health SOS: The Shadow Side of the Wireless Revolution,* 110 Questions on Electromagnetic Pollution from a Forum at the Commonwealth Club of California. Diagram created by Electriclean. Further reading: *Bibliography of Reported Biological Phenomena (Effects) and Clinical Manifestations attributed to Microwave and Radio-Frequency.*

22. *Electromagnetic Fields and the Life Environment,* Mahra K, Musil J, Tuha H, Institute of Industrial Hygiene and Industrial Diseases, Prague. Translated from the Czech. San Francisco Press Inc., Berkeley CA USA.

23. Diagram created by Electriclean. Further reading: Bibliography of Reported *Biological Phenomena (Effects) and Clinical Manifestations attributed to Microwave and Radio-Frequency Radiation,* Zorach R Glaser, PhD, LT, MSC, USNR Research Report, Project MF12.524.015-00043, Report No.2, Naval Medical Research Institute, National Naval Medical Center, Bethesda, Maryland 20014, USA. Second printing with revisions, corrections and additions: 20 April 1972. More than 2000 references on the biological responses to radio frequency and microwave radiation, published up to June 1971, are included in the bibliography.

CHAPTER 10

1. Some guidelines are even higher.

2. There would possibly be many more variables, such as the type of magnetic fields that are present and the assessment of the plumbing environment, etc.

3. To address all the frequencies and fields from 0Hz to 300 GHz is a vast area.

4. Information is taken from the Expert Testimony of Dr Magda Havas submitted February 9, 2009, *Report to the Workplace Safety and Insurance Appeals Tribunal Breast Cancer and Occupational Exposure to Electromagnetic Fields Response,* November 18, 2008 and Response to Request from Heidi Evelyn, Tribunal Counsel Office, Workplace Safety and Insurance Appeals Tribunal, Dated: January 7 & 9, 2009.

   (Author's note: Cancer promoters have major implications for the incidence of cancer because they increase the number of cases of cancer that become evident. We are always developing small cancers that are recognized by our immune system and destroyed. Any factor that increases the growth rate of these small cancers gives them an advantage over the immune system, and as a result more people develop clinical cancers that require treatment. The concurrent effect of the promotion of cancer-cell growth and the increase in the malignant characteristics of these cells leads to an increased incidence of cancers with faster-than-normal rates of growth).

CHAPTER 11

1. Havas M, Rae W, Tel-Oren A, Ecopolitan.com 2009 – www.ecopolitan.com/healthresources/emfprotection/147-health-effects-radio

2. Excerpted from Dr Robert O Becker, *Cross Currents: The Perils of Electropollution, The Promise of Electromedicine,* 1990 pp 206-207.

CHAPTER 12

1. Further reading: www.iaea.org/Publications/Magazines Bulletin/Bull502/50205813137.html

2. BMJ 2013; 347:15193 doi:10.1136/bmj.f5193

3. Wertheimer N, Leeper E, *Electrical Wiring Configurations and Childhood Cancer, Am J of Epidemiol.* Vol 109 (3): pp 273-284, 1979.

4. Savitz *et al. Case-control Study of Childhood Cancer and Exposure to 60-Hz Magnetic Fields, Am J of Epidemiol.* Vol 128, No 1, 1988.

5. Wertheimer N, Leeper E, *Adult cancer related to electrical wires near the home, Int J Epidemiol.* 1982; 11:345-55.

6. Erren T, in Stevens, Wilson, Anderson, 1977, p 729.

7. Genuis SJ, p 6.

8. Australian TV program – Nine with David and Kim – August 7, 2007.

9. Rafnsson V, et al., *Risk of Breast Cancer in Female Flight Attendants: A Population-Based Study* (Iceland), *Cancer Causes and Control* 12, no: 2 (2001): 95-101, doi: 10.1023/A:1008983416836.

10. Carlo G and Schram M, *Cell Phones: Invisible Hazards in the Wireless Age.*

CHAPTER 13

1. GS filters are tuned capacitors that reduce high frequencies voltages (transients) on electrical wires. They protect sensitive electronic equipment. Research shows they also reduce symptoms of electrohypersensitivity. These filters need to be installed with proper monitoring (microsurge meter) to ensure levels are sufficiently low for maximum benefit (visit www.getpurepower.ca for dirty electricity meters and GS filters). Source: www.magdahavas.com – April 3, 2004

PART 2: LIGHT THAT HEALS

1. Hyperthermic Oncology 1984 Review Lectures, Symposium. *Summaries & Workshop Summaries*, Overgaard J, ed., Taylor & Francis, London & Philadelphia. Proceedings of the 4th International Symposium, on Hyperthermic Oncology, held at Aarhus, Denmark, 2-6 July 1984, Vol 2, 1985, p 199-209.

2. Oschman JL, p 95. After Guyton 1991, with kind permission of WB Saunders Co.

3. Chernet BT, Levin M, *Transmembrane voltage potential is an essential cellular parameter for the detection and control of tumor development in a Xenopus model.* Dis. Model. Mech. 8 February doi:10.1242/dmm.010835 Article

Bioelectric signals can be used to detect early cancer. http://medicalxpress.com/news/2013-02-bioelectric-early-cancer.html

4. Gerber R, p 416.

5. Becker RO, p 140.

6. Milham S, 2010 p 1. Article, *Medical Hypotheses* doi:10.1016/jmehy.2010.01.033.

7. Personal discussions with PowerTube inventor, Martin Frischknecht.

8. Personal correspondence with Dr Randy Beck.

9. Research paper first published in the *International Journal of Medical Sciences* 2010; 7 (1): 29-35. Full paper available at www.medsci.org/v07p0029.pdf.

10. Philips A & J, Positive Effects of EMFs http://www.powerwatch.org.uk/library/downloads/positive-emfs-1-cancer-2012-04.pdf.

11. Oschman JL, p 74.

12. www.magdahavas.com/dr-oz-on-pemf-therapy-and-pain-control/

13. Professors Morgan G, Royal North Shore, Ward R, Prince of Wales and Barton M, Liverpool Hospital oncologists and radiotherapists of Sydney, conducted a study in 2004 regarding the debate on the funding and availability of cytotoxic drugs. The aim of the study was to answer questions about the contribution of curative or adjvant cycotoxic chemotherapy to survival in adult cancer patients.

14. The advantage of local hyperthermia combined with conformal radiotherapy should be confirmed by a randomized phase 3 trial, comparing irradiation plus androgen suppression therapy with or without hyperthermia. *International Journal of Hyperthermia* 2007, 148 vol 23 no 5, pp 451-456 PMID: 17701536.

15. Dr Jacobi van der Zee's paper titled *Part 1: Clinical Hyperthermia* was reviewed in the *International Journal of Hyperthermia* March 2008 and presented at the Kadota Fund International Conference.

16. Very Weak RF Signals Show Promise for Treating Inoperable Liver Cancer – Dose Is 100-1,000 times lower than from a cell phone, August 15, 2011 – www.microwavenews.com

17. Source: www.novocure.com

18. *With Electrical Stimulation to the Spinal Cord, Paralyzed Man Walks Again –* www.foxnews.com/scitech/2011/05/20electrical-stimulation-spinal-cord-paralyzed-man-walks

19. Georgetown University Medical Center (GUMC), Washington DC. www.hippocrates.com.au/Hippocrates-news-archive/vitamin-ditem/375-viamin-d-and-reduced-breast-cancer.

20. *New research suggests vitamin D status is a predictor of disability and death*

after stroke event, Tu W *et al,* Serum 25-hydroxyvitamin D predicts the short-term outcomes of Chinese patients with acute ischaemic stroke. Clinical science 2014. Vitamin D Council, December 11, 2013 post.

21. Liberman J, p 140.

22. Liberman J, p 143-144.

23. Oschman JL, p 88.

24. *NASA Light Technology Successfully Reduces Cancer Patients Painful Side Effects from Radiation and Chemotherapy. HEALS Device for Cancer Treatment, Wound Healing, and Pain Management Light therapy helps fight cancer and provides natural, drug-free pain relief.*

25. Sourced from: www.bioptron.com and conversations with a therapist.

26. Information sourced from: www.sensolite.hu/en/.

27. Liberman J, p 115.

28. Personal conversations with company doctor in Australia, information from the company's PowerPoint presentations supplied and information sourced from www.ngpdt.com.

29. Liberman J, p 111.

30. Liberman J, p 189.

31. Myss C, p 35.

32. Liberman J, p 132.

33. lighting.philips.com.

34. Liberman J, p 104-105.

35. Whitcroft J, KeyRight PowerPoint presentation.

36. Liberman J, p 159-161.

37. Gerber R, p 339-344.

38. Gerber R, p 339-344.

39. Gerber R, p 339-344.

40. Gerber R, p 339-344.

41. Gerber R, p 339-344.

42. Oschman JL, p 129.

43. Gerber R, p 365.

EPILOGUE

1. Neophytou C, p 356.

2. Liberman J, Foreword.

3. Shealy CN and Myss CM, p 167. The Ukrainian nuclear physicists claim that the cells of each organ collectively project a stream of gigahertz energy along the path or vector of least resistance to some point on the surface of the body at the base of a finger or toenail with flow to and from this point. Quantum physicists report that the Sun bathes the Earth with 52-78 GHz energy, among others, at one ten-billionth of a watt/cm^2.

4. Tesla detected the electric scalar wave and Meyl the magnetic scalar wave.

5. Oschman JL, p 206.

6. Oschman JL, p 177.

7. www.tompaladinoscalarenergy.com

8. Scalar energy is longitudinal and recent research has shown DNA generates a longitudinal wave.

   The magnetic scalar wave, as an aspect of the neutrinos and therefore being quicker than light, is used in all biology. Meyl explains how the DNA is sending information and energy as an antenna using a DNA wave – Tesla Scalar Waves and the Unified Field Theory. Meyl K, in *Cellular Communication by Magnetic Scalar Waves* states:

   > The DNA generates a longitudinal wave which propagates within the magnetic field vector ... Magnetic scalar wave theory explains how the dual base pair-stored information of the genetic code is formed. The process of converting electrical modulation into 'piggyback' information that transfers or is sent from the cell nucleus to another cell is a revolutionary theory. Information transferred at the receiving end during the reverse process takes place involving a change in the physical and chemical cellular structure. The energy required to power the chemical process, is now understood by the extended field theory to come from the magnetic scalar wave.

   Note: Further information is available at: Prof Meyl detected DNA-wave and scalar wave technology Henning Witte http://vimeo.com/41763071. Also refer to Meyl K, *DNA and Cell Resonance*. The video, *The Healing Universe*, by physicist John Michael Mallon, explains scalar energy in more simple terms.

INDEX

Nm 174, 176
Non-ionizing radiation 52, 55, 68-69, 85, 93, 102, 104, 106, 110, 121, 128, 132
Non-linear 14, 198
Non-thermal effects 66, 80, 93, 166
Norway 103-104
Novocure 170-171
NovoTTF-100A 170-171

O'Leary, C 85
O'Connor, E 63
Obesity 23, 48
Ohio 23, 88
Oncothermia 167-168
Ontario 34, 74-75, 125
Oschman, JL 15, 108, 160, 161, 195, 196, 198
Oscilloscope 40, 205-206
Ossiander, EM 22
Ott, J 42, 197
Oxidative stress 90-91, 105, 108

Pacemakers 82, 162, 164, 172
Pain 13, 16, 26, 43, 46, 71, 76, 82, 100, 112, 124, 154-155, 159, 161-164, 168-169, 172, 179-182, 185
Palpitations 71
Pancreatic 102
Parcells, H 194
Parry, B 195
Pasche, B 168-170
Patnick, J 56
PAVE PAWS 61
PDT 186-189
PEA 81
PEMF 160-162, 164
PER 2000 163-164
Periodontal 183, 186
Pert, C 193
Pharoah, P 56
PHz 176
Photobiomodulation 177
Photons 175, 180
Photosensitizer 186, 188-189
Pineal gland 24, 91-92, 120
Pituitary gland 24, 196
Polarized 143, 183-185
Positron meter 34, 205
Powerwatch 67, 95

Pregnant 15, 29, 39, 44, 89, 91-93, 100, 102, 117, 174
Premenstrual syndrome 195
Project Pandora 60
Proliferation 93, 95, 97-98, 150, 170, 175
Prostate 23, 58, 61, 63, 93, 102, 104, 123, 169, 183, 189, 191, 195
Proton Beam Therapy 172

Quartz 143, 195-196, 199

Rad 55
Radar 60, 61, 62, 64, 77, 86, 97, 106, 114
Radiation 16, 26, 29, 31, 35, 39, 42, 48, 50-52, 55-58, 60-66, 68-77, 79-81, 84-86, 89, 92-98, 102, 104-107, 109-110, 113, 115, 117, 121-123, 128-130, 133, 135-137, 142, 152, 154, 164-166, 168-171, 179-180, 184-185, 191, 202
Radiowave Therapy Research Institute 167
Rea, W 14, 49, 135
Rapid Aging Syndrome 46
Rau, T 161
Receptor 58, 119, 120
Rehani, M 129
Reproductive 24, 27, 53, 60, 62, 82, 92, 108
Resnik, V 44
Resonance 108, 142-143, 146-147, 166, 179, 197
Resonance-magnetic 26, 83, 120
Resonance- nuclear magnetic 164
Rett syndrome 90
RF EMF 45, 55, 57, 62-63, 67, 77, 96, 100, 102, 104, 114-116, 131
Richards, D 152
Rife, RR 142143, 192
RNA 16, 26, 87, 175, 181
Roder, D 53
Rouleaux index 163, 178
Russia 38, 44, 60, 68, 154, 158, 168
Russian 30, 32, 38, 60, 66, 68-69, 84, 96, 109, 116, 142, 158-159, 175, 177, 186

SAD 175
Salamander 144
Salford, L 65,
Salivary gland 55
San Diego 54, 118, 133, 173
Sanskrit 193, 196

ABOUT THE AUTHOR

Donna Fisher loves a challenge and her very first one came early. At the tender age of four, like millions of children worldwide she started school. Having stuttered on every letter since she first spoke, reading in class was torture. Stuttering can become so serious that it makes a vocational failure of even a talented person, but not in Donna's case. She overcame her disordered speech after years of effort and today her stutter is mild and infrequent. She asserts, with great determination, that she will gain complete fluency.

After leaving school Donna involved herself in many worthy causes and successful commercial enterprises, but it wasn't enough to satisfy her drive, energy and restlessness. After studying transpersonal psychology, she attended an intensive workshop on leadership and went on to complete a thesis with special emphasis on the positive role of women in co-creating a better world.

In 1999 the first letter from the electric utility company arrived alerting her to the issue of the invisible fields from electricity being a concern. Donna's increasing comprehension of owning her own mind combined easily with her patient nature, leading her to study the attributes of the 'Warrior Path' and the ways in which change can come through peaceful means. Shortly after that Donna began working in a voluntary capacity for a non-profit association dealing with child abuse for 18 months.

When Donna took on the case against the power company she had long learned that the way forward for all of personkind is through sharing reality in a co-creative way, and the way forward for her personally was by intervening with positive action on issues that were particularly important to her. She believes that by claiming and owning one's mind humanity can live intelligently through the heart. While a little knowledge can be dangerous too much knowledge takes away the heart sense.

Born in Australia, Donna has grown a wide following through her many international lectures and her website donnafisher.net. While there is a touch of the crusader in Donna this energetic person does not invade your privacy but encourages you, albeit with great passion to first, do no harm.

ALSO BY DONNA FISHER

Read the exciting account of the author and her neighbours in *Silent Fields – the Growing Cancer Cluster Story: When Electricity Kills*. With little technical, medical and legal experience they battled with a large public power company to stop them from building an electricity substation and an installation of powerlines very close to their homes which they felt would be unsafe. Follow this courageous band of dedicated and committed people through red-tape, bureaucracy, disinterested politicians and the courts as they challenge the biggest corporation in town in a quest to save lives.

This landmark case may reveal one of the biggest public health scandals in Australia. Donna Fisher's book marked the beginning of her efforts to expose world-wide EMF issues to the public.

Limited Edition paperback available at: **donnafisher.net**

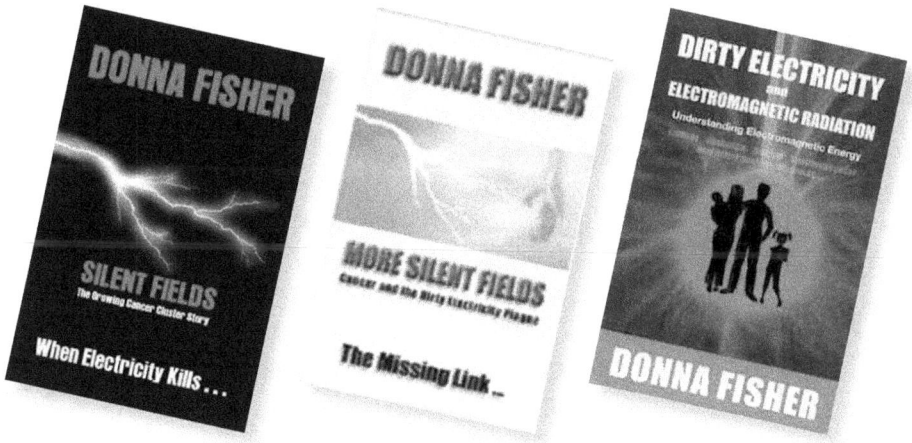

www.ingramcontent.com/pod-product-compliance
Lightning Source LLC
Chambersburg PA
CBHW070403270326
41926CB00014B/2678